art therapy for every day

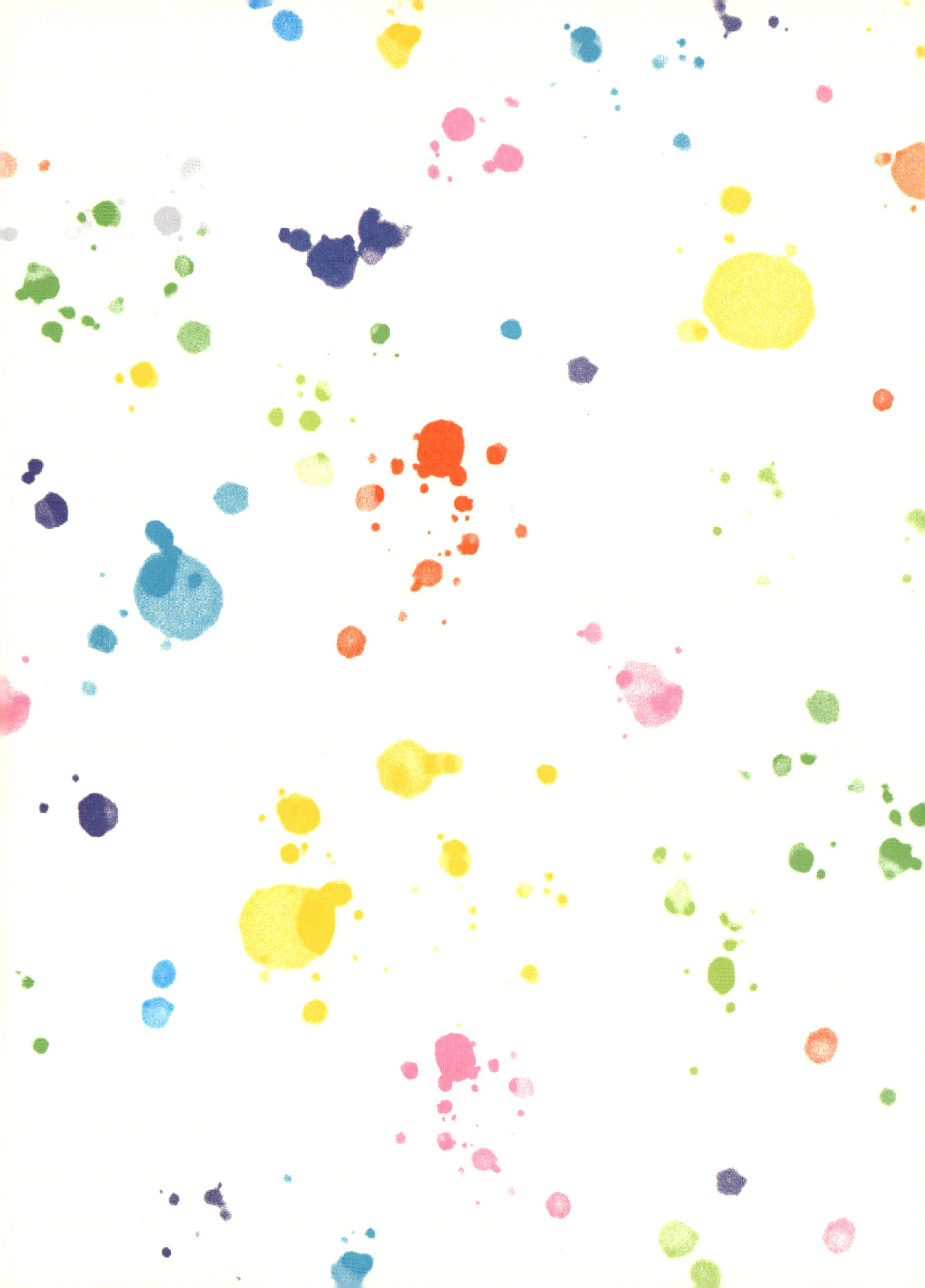

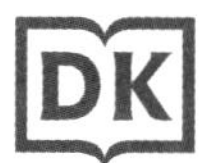

Nadia Paredes
MA, LMFT, ATR

art therapy for every day

365 tools & exercises to help you create, heal & grow

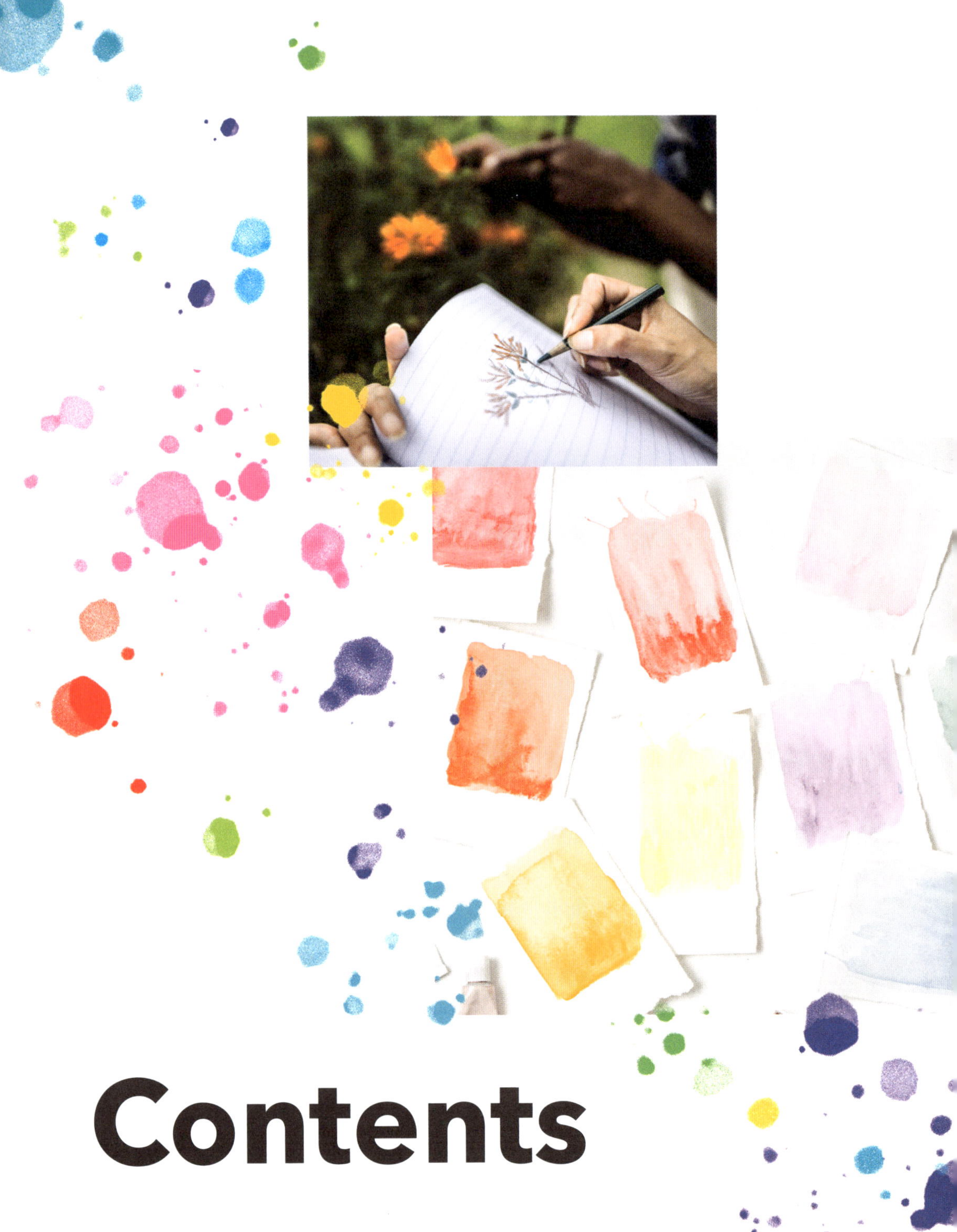

Contents

Introduction

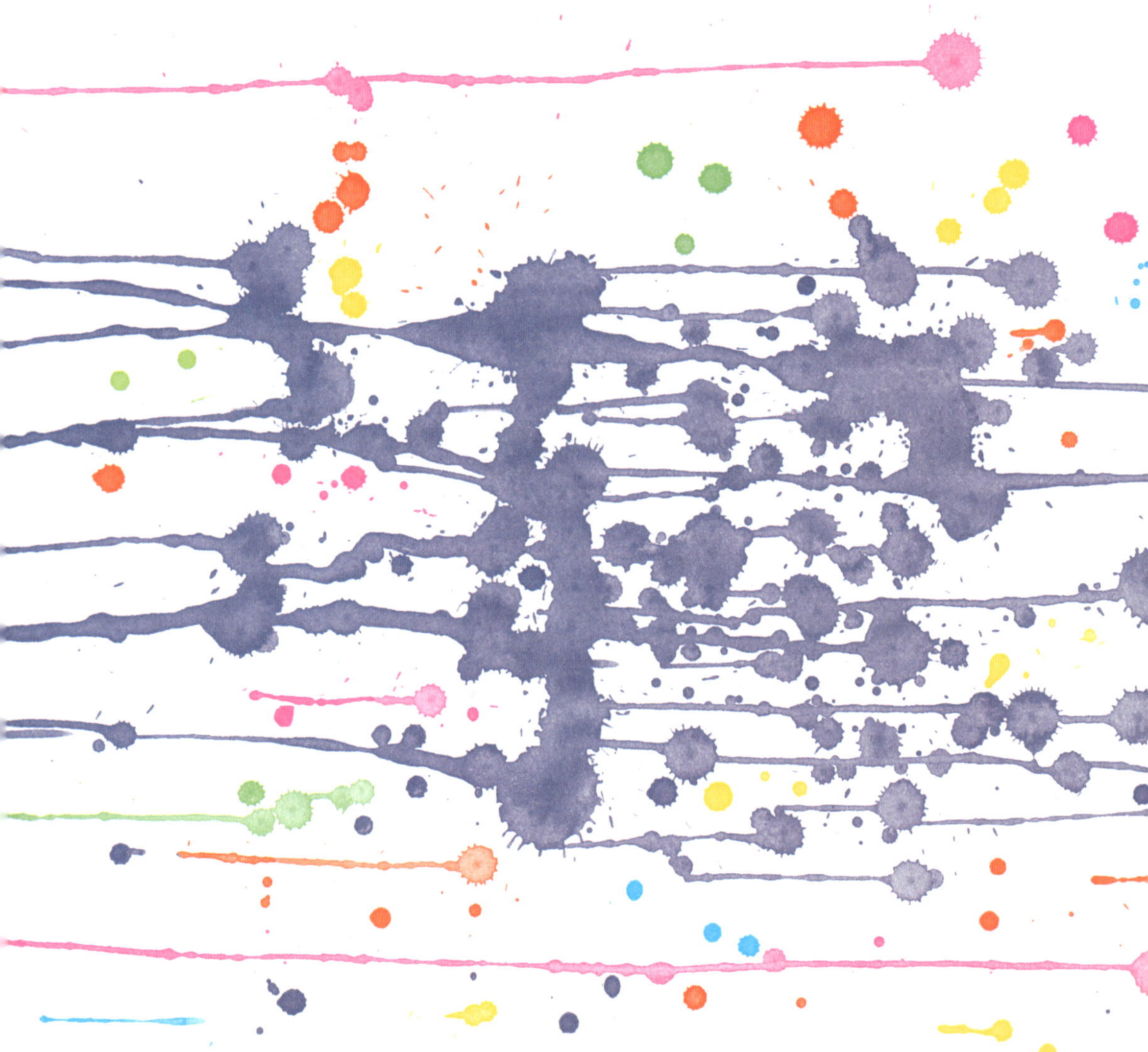

We are all born with the ability and the need to create. As the American actress, Phylicia Rashad, famously said, "Before a child speaks, it sings. Before they write, they paint. As soon as they stand, they dance. Art is the basis of human expression." However, life can get in the way, and we often lose connection with our innate creativity. This book will help awaken your dormant inner artist.

Art is powerful medicine. By regularly tapping into your creativity and expressing your inner world, you can develop meaningful tools to help you understand yourself better, process your emotions and experiences, and navigate life's challenges. You don't need to have any special talent or training – just a willingness to connect and bring forth what's already inside.

I am an art therapist, a certified intuitive painting facilitator, and a mindfulness specialist, and I have designed the exercises in this book using techniques that are backed by psychology and personally proven in my own practice. Within these pages, I hope you will find many ways to connect with your creative side, increase your self-knowledge, and improve your emotional health and general wellbeing.

What is art therapy?

Before we get started, it's important to understand the differences between art therapy and therapeutic art. Both offer benefits, but differ in approach – think of them as opposite ends of a creative healing spectrum, with this book positioned somewhere between the two.

- Art therapy is a recognized mental health profession – an art therapist is professionally trained and will have an art and psychology background. Therapeutic art is something you can do by yourself or with others, without needing to have psychological knowledge to benefit.
- Art therapy combines science-based psychological approaches with an understanding of how the different properties of art materials and practices affect the mind, enabling art therapists to tailor methods and mediums to client needs. Therapeutic art involves general knowledge and experimentation with art-making.
- Art therapy typically addresses a defined issue, such as managing a specific mental health condition or offering education related to emotional coping skills. In contrast, therapeutic art doesn't require a particular goal and may contribute to an overall sense of wellbeing.

While this book provides an invaluable creative outlet using techniques proven to be beneficial for your health and happiness, it is not a substitute for professional mental health care. If you feel overwhelmed and find you are having difficulties navigating your everyday life, seek support from someone you trust or a qualified professional.

How to use this book...

I designed this book using preventive mental health techniques, applying my in-depth knowledge about psychological health, mindfulness, and art methods and materials to make art more accessible and inclusive. Its purpose is to support your mental wellbeing goals by providing tools to improve your emotional health and overcome self-limiting beliefs. However, as you will be guiding yourself through these pages, it serves as a therapeutic art book.

Each chapter offers art exercises designed to encourage self-reflection and support your wellbeing. After each activity, a series of follow-up questions deepens your creative process by making space for self-reflection. The exercises vary in length so that they fit easily into your daily schedule, and within each chapter you'll find a series of related exercises to be completed in a single session for when you want to dig deeper and focus on a certain goal.

The beauty of art is that it provides a means to record and observe changes in our internal development. Make sure you always have a journal at hand to note down your discoveries and track your thoughts and feelings; you can also revisit any of the exercises at a later date to see if your perspective changes over time. Remember that these exercises are guides for personal growth and healing – there are no right or wrong answers, just opportunities for greater self-awareness.

It's not always easy to recognize or articulate what we are feeling. To guide you through your art therapy journey, I've created a list of core values and emotions to help you identify yours. The values list is inspired by Brené Brown, a renowned research professor in the field of personal development, and the emotions are based on the Hoffman Process, an international programme offering personal transformational work.

Core values and emotions

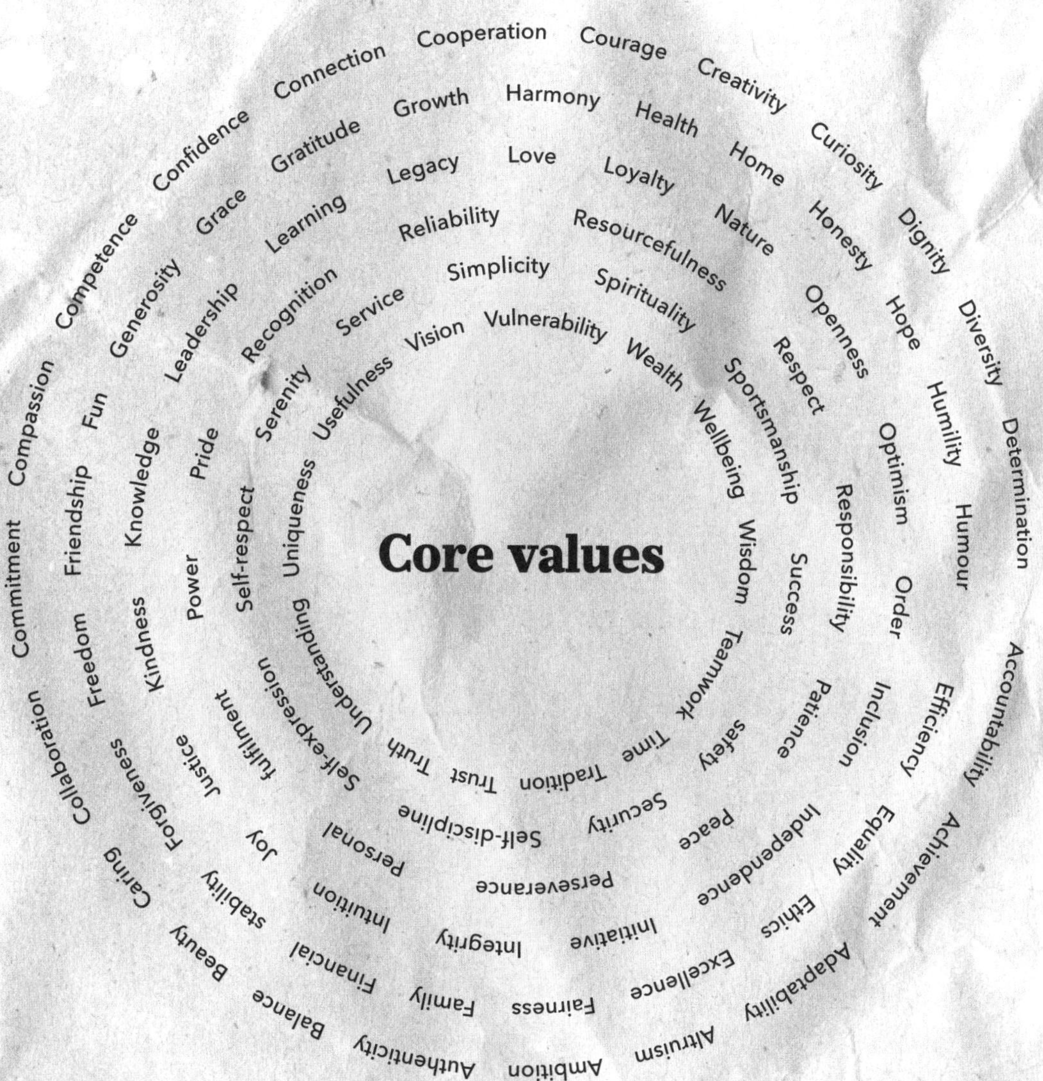

Core values
Cooperation Courage Creativity
Connection Growth Harmony Health Curiosity
Confidence Gratitude Legacy Love Home Dignity
Grace Learning Reliability Loyalty Honesty Diversity
Competence Generosity Recognition Simplicity Resourcefulness Nature Openness Humility Determination
Compassion Leadership Serenity Service Spirituality Respect Hope Humour Accountability
Fun Knowledge Self-respect Vision Vulnerability Wealth Sportsmanship Optimism Order
Commitment Friendship Power Pride Uniqueness Usefulness Wellbeing Wisdom Success Responsibility Inclusion Efficiency
Freedom Kindness Self-expression Teamwork Patience Independence Equality Achievement
Collaboration Forgiveness Justice fulfilment Understanding Truth Trust Time Tradition Safety Security Peace Ethics Adaptability
Caring Joy Intuition Personal Self-discipline Perseverance Initiative Excellence Altruism
Beauty stability Financial Family Fairness
Balance Authenticity Ambition

Emotions

Anger

Agitated
Bitter
Frustrated
Hostile
Irritated
Upset
Vindictive

Sadness

Disappointed
Discouraged
Gloomy
Grief
Heartbroken
Hopeless
Lonely
Unhappy

Fear

Afraid
Anxious
Apprehensive
Nervous
Panicky
Paralyzed
Scared
Terrified
Worried

Guilt

Regretful
Remorseful

Stressed

Burnt out
Cranky
Edgy
Exhausted
Overwhelmed
Rattled
Shaken
Tense
Worn out

Powerful

Brave
Capable
Confident
Proud
Worthy

Joy

Amazed
Awestruck
Blissful
Enchanted
Energized
Excited
Happy
Playful
Rejuvenated
Satisfied

Doubt

Apprehensive
Dissatisfied
Hesitant
Questioning
Rejecting
Shocked
Sceptical

Accepting

Calm
Centred
Fulfilled
Grounded
Relaxed

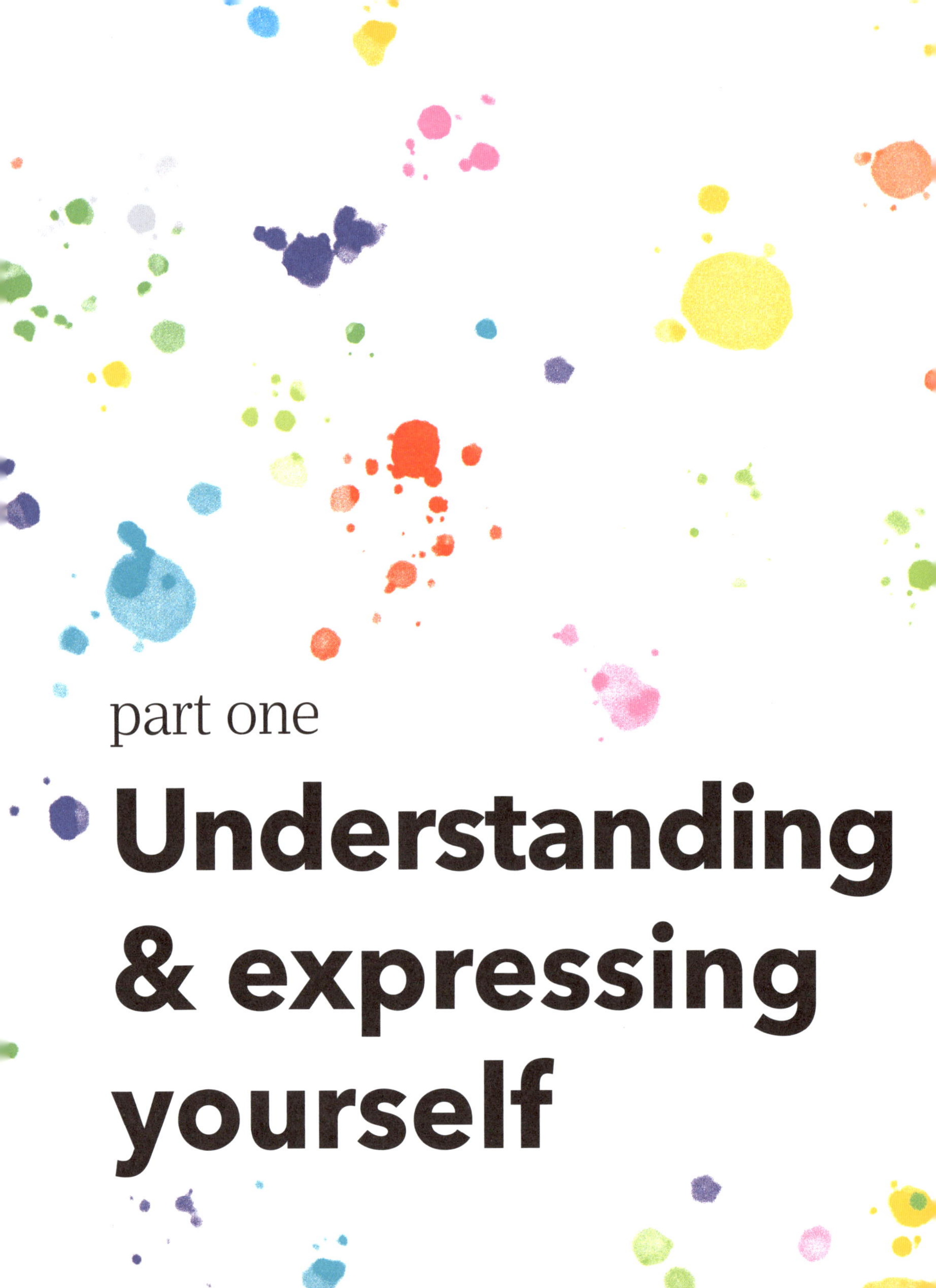
part one
Understanding
& expressing
yourself

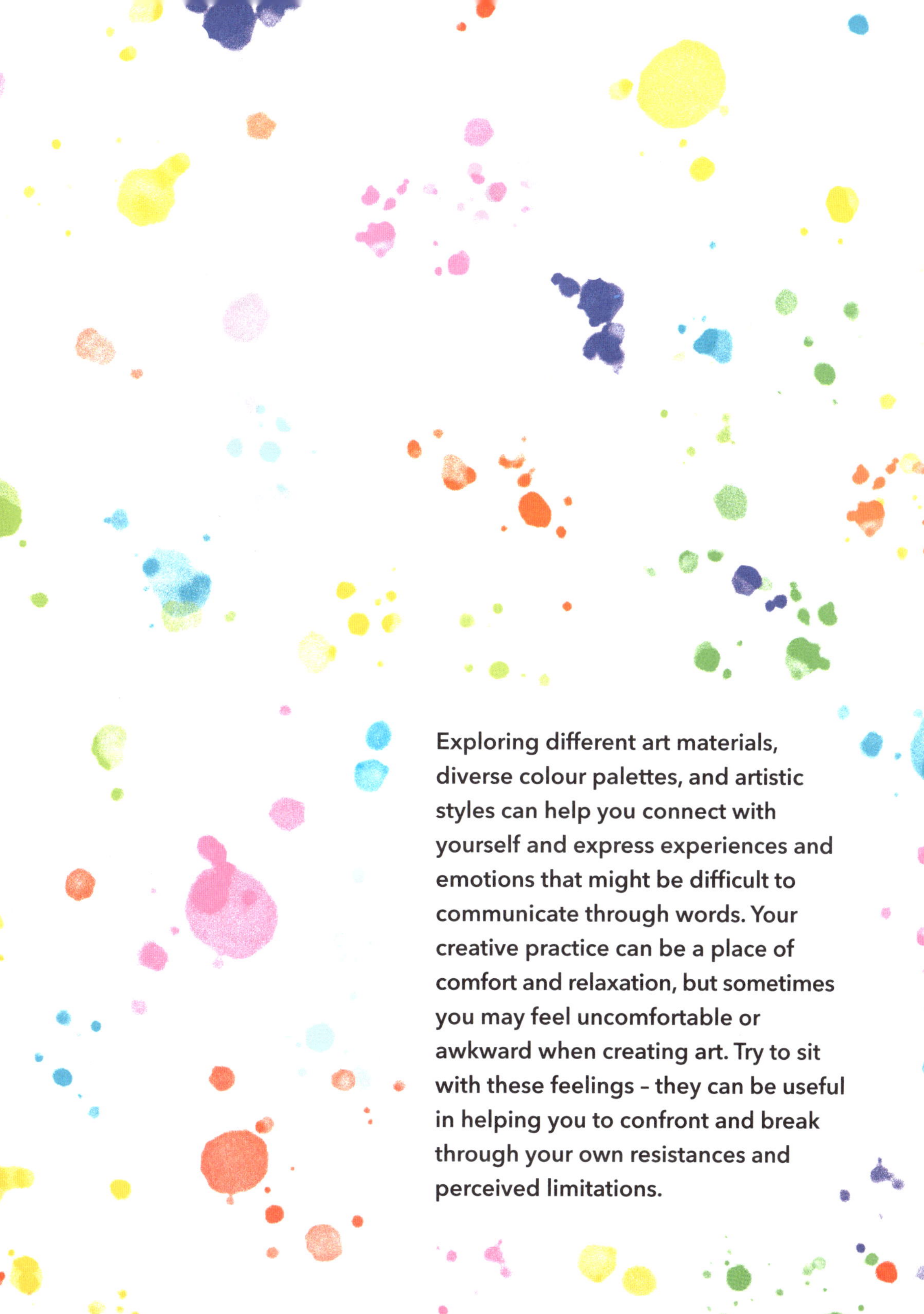

Exploring different art materials, diverse colour palettes, and artistic styles can help you connect with yourself and express experiences and emotions that might be difficult to communicate through words. Your creative practice can be a place of comfort and relaxation, but sometimes you may feel uncomfortable or awkward when creating art. Try to sit with these feelings – they can be useful in helping you to confront and break through your own resistances and perceived limitations.

Finding your way in

Since ancient times, humans have used art to heal and connect. Today, art therapy continues this tradition by blending creativity with neuroscience. The healing arts aren't about perfection, they are about expression, so step outside of your critical mind and explore with colour and movement, allowing your inner world to emerge. Focus on the process, not the product, because ultimately that is what matters on this journey.

001

Testing out colour palettes

Try this when
you want to explore your emotional landscape

You will need
Paper, watercolours, mixing palette, paintbrushes

30 minutes

Divide a sheet of paper into 12 squares, then fill the squares with four different colour schemes – for example brights, dark tones, light tints, or black and white. Observe which colour values are calling your attention. Are you able to just choose one?

SELF-REFLECTION Were you surprised by your choices? Why? Do specific colour schemes mean something to you? Do you prefer certain colours because you have associated them with a particular mood?

002

What does this colour palette mean?

Try this when
you want to deepen your emotional awareness

You will need
Previously created colour palette, paper, pen, pencils

20 minutes

Place the colour palette you created in the previous exercise in front of you. Look at the individual schemes and identify five feelings they each evoke (see pp.10–13 for inspiration). When you are done, notice what feelings come to you as you considered each palette and write down your obervations. Once you have figured out what emotions you associate with different colours, try using them intentionally to evoke a particular feeling.

SELF-REFLECTION Do you recognize a trend? Which feeling surprised you the most? What do these feelings reveal about your current emotional state?

003

The colour story

Try this when
you can't find the words to
express your emotions

You will need
Previously created colour
palette, paper, paintbrushes

15 minutes

Look at the colour palette you created in the first
exercise and think about a significant positive
memory or life experience. Express it on the page
using just colours and abstract shapes, no words or
recognizable images. Let the colours tell the story.

SELF-REFLECTION What colours did you choose and
why? Notice if any colours dominated the scene.
Do you have a special connection with them in your
everyday life? What does this reveal about the way
you emotionally connect with colour?

004

Black or colour?

Try this when
you want to explore your
comfort zones

You will need
Paper, black marker,
coloured markers

15 minutes

Create a drawing using only black lines and shapes.
Now recreate the drawing using different colours
that aren't black. Notice the difference in how each
iteration makes you feel.

SELF-REFLECTION Do you prefer one drawing over the
other? If you choose the black rendering, could this
mean you are looking for predictability and stability
in your life? Or did you choose the coloured
drawing? If so, might this indicate that you are
seeking more stimulation and diversity?

REMEMBER You can try this exercise at different times
in your life and see how your perspective changes.

005

Colour as a self-portrait

Try this when
you want to connect with
your authentic self

You will need
Paper, coloured pencils

15 minutes

Draw an abstract self-portrait using just
colours and shapes to represent your
personality or inner world. Forget about
realistic skin tones or facial features
– focus on what colours express you best.

SELF-REFLECTION Which colours feel most
connected to you, and why? Did you use
any colours you don't normally associate
with yourself? What could this self-portrait
be revealing about how you see yourself?

Colour in art therapy

Exploring colour in art therapy
allows us to deepen our
understanding of our own
expressive visual language.
By recognizing personal colour
preferences and their meanings,
we can connect more
authentically to our emotions
and experiences. Colours can
also serve as a powerful tool
for metaphorical expression,
expanding our creative language
and providing new ways to
communicate feelings that may
be difficult to put into words.
Understanding our personal
palette can enhance self-
awareness and make artistic
expression an even more
meaningful and intuitive process.

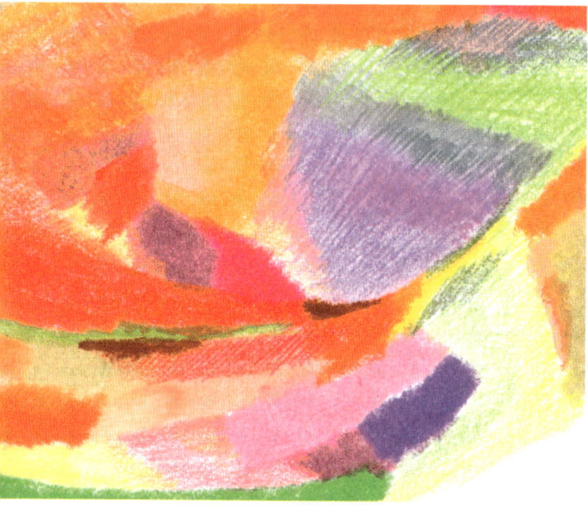

Testing out materials

Noticing how different parts of you connect with various art media can help you learn what your body and mind find calming or stressful. This awareness is useful when trying to regulate your emotions. We are all wired differently, and some people feel a stronger connection to their body, while others are more attuned to their mind or emotions.

Try this when
you want to understand yourself better

1 hour 30 minutes

006 Exploring rigid materials

You will need

Paper, pencils, markers

Experiment with different coloured pencils or markers by scribbling, drawing, and playing around with colour. Give yourself 5 minutes per material to test out each one.

007 Exploring fluid materials

You will need

Three pieces of paper, watercolours, paintbrushes

Now, using a paintbrush, cover a page with paint. Take another piece of paper and first wet it, then again fill it with paint. On a third piece of paper, use your fingers to cover it with paint. Allow 5 minutes to try out each application.

008 Exploring unconventional materials

You will need

Paper, coffee, tea, wine

Art shouldn't just be about using conventional materials. Next, test coffee, tea, and wine, on a sheet of paper for 5 minutes, then think about your experience.

009 **Exploring 3D art-making**

You will need

Paperclips, Play-Doh

As you might already know, art is not only created in two dimensions. Last, allow yourself 5 minutes to make a sculpture with paperclips and Play-Doh, then reflect on your experience.

SELF-REFLECTION When you have finished exploring each material, write down your reactions (physical, emotional, and rational) using the template below.

material	body	feelings	thoughts

What materials did you prefer? Which did you reject? Did you notice a feeling of calm with a specific material? Or did a material make you feel uncomfortable? What does this tell you about your own comfort zones and creative boundaries? Can you identify which materials soothe you? Try using the more uncomfortable ones to help push yourself out of your comfort zones safely.

010

Small and big format

Try this when
you want to understand
your comfort zones

You will need
Three pieces of paper,
pencil

15 minutes

Look around your house for a simple object that you
wish to draw. On the first piece of paper, draw the
object as small as a coin. Then, on the second piece
of paper, draw it to completely fill the page. Last, on
the third sheet, draw it at a medium size.

SELF-REFLECTION What size felt more comfortable to
you? Could the size be reflective of how much space
you are willing to take up in the world? In what areas
of your life do you feel most comfortable taking up
space, and where do you tend to hold back?

011

Thick or thin

Try this when
you want to explore your
personal boundaries

You will need
Paper, paint,
paintbrushes

5 minutes

Exploring size can help you understand how you set
boundaries – both physical and emotional. Lay down
some thick and thin lines by varying the pressure of
your paintbrush. In a single stroke, see how many
variations you can achieve. Fill one area of a page
with thick lines and another with thin lines. Notice
which line quality feels most natural or soothing.

SELF-REFLECTION Which type of line did you feel the
most drawn to? How might this reflect your current
approach to personal boundaries? Could favouring
thicker lines suggest a need for strong boundaries,
or does preferring thinner lines indicate a need for
more flexibility?

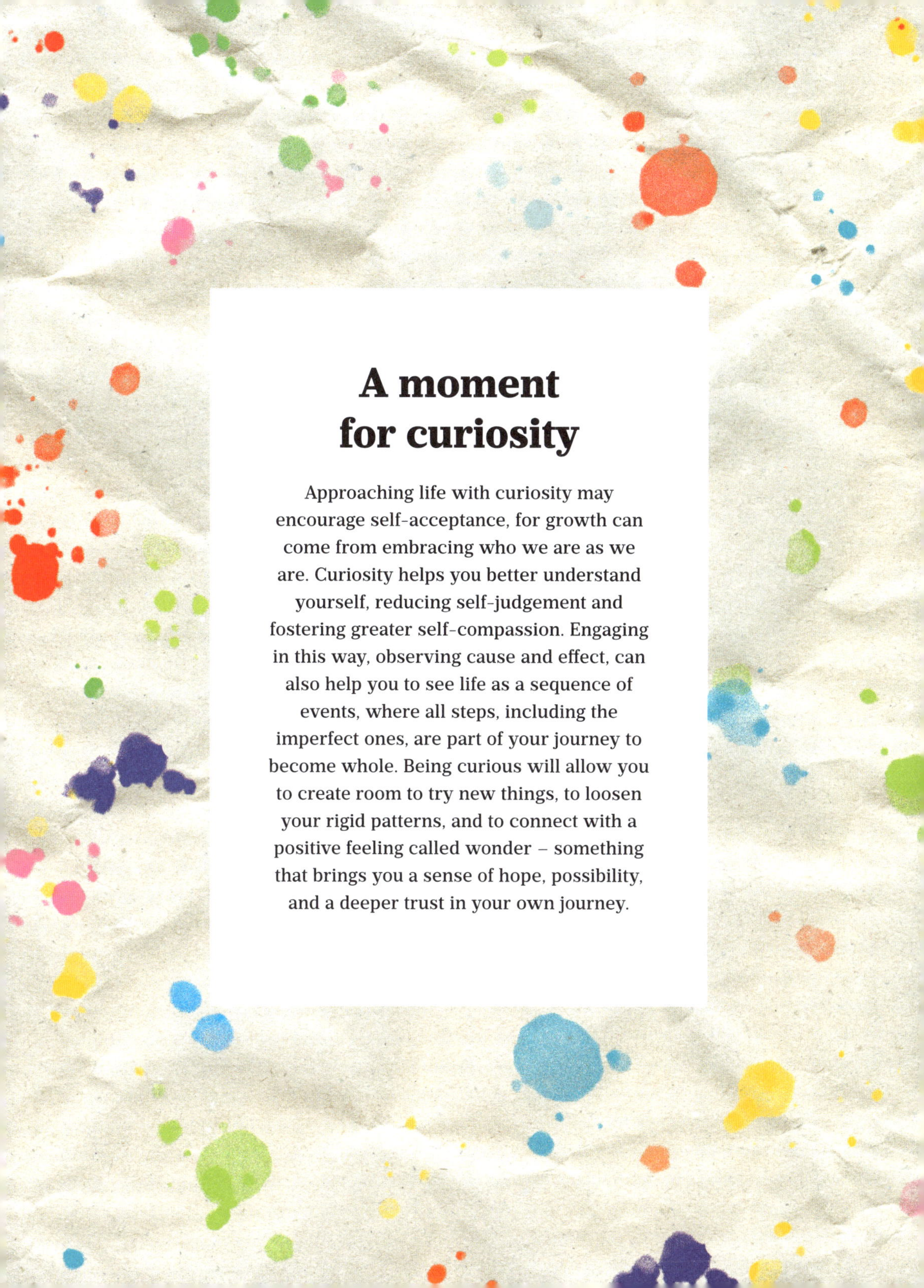

A moment for curiosity

Approaching life with curiosity may encourage self-acceptance, for growth can come from embracing who we are as we are. Curiosity helps you better understand yourself, reducing self-judgement and fostering greater self-compassion. Engaging in this way, observing cause and effect, can also help you to see life as a sequence of events, where all steps, including the imperfect ones, are part of your journey to become whole. Being curious will allow you to create room to try new things, to loosen your rigid patterns, and to connect with a positive feeling called wonder – something that brings you a sense of hope, possibility, and a deeper trust in your own journey.

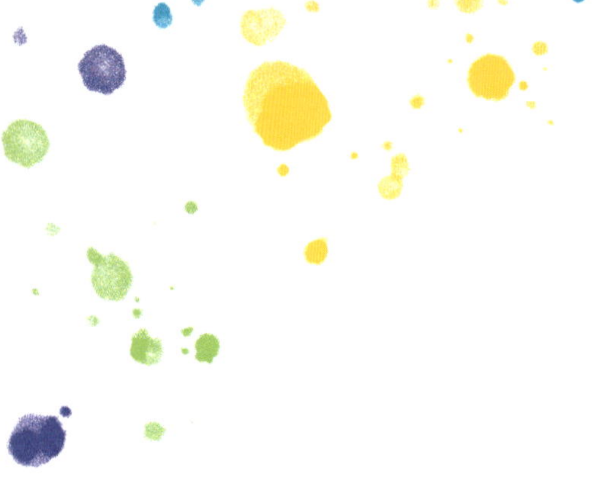

012

Speed art

Try this when
you want to explore your
relationship with time

You will need
Paper, pencil, timer

5 minutes

Divide a piece of paper into 16 squares and draw a
triangle inside each. When you are done, set a timer
for 45 seconds, then try to draw as many things as
you can using a triangle as the base of each drawing.
Could one become a tree? A piece of pizza? You
figure it out.

SELF-REFLECTION How did limiting the time affect your
creativity? Was it better to do it without thinking, or did
you feel under pressure and unproductive? What does
this say about your own need for time now? Could you
do with slowing down and finding your own rhythm?

013

City sculpture

Try this when
you want to explore new
ways to see your world

You will need
Everyday objects around
your house, paper, pencil

30 minutes

Use this exercise to dive into your own beliefs about
the art world and how they may limit your ability to
create expressively. Using objects you find around
your home, build a cityscape. Use medicine bottles,
glassware, and cereal boxes. When complete, draw
the city skyline on a piece of paper.

SELF-REFLECTION Were you able to find inspiration
in everyday objects to create art? Or did you struggle
to believe that this composition could be called
artistic? Why?

014

Found-textures collage

Try this when
you want to connect more
deeply with your feelings

You will need
Paper, coloured pencils,
scissors, glue

30 minutes

Exploring textures in art helps you
channel curiosity and connect with your
emotions, revealing comfort, tension, or
resistance. It can help you to experience
the world using all of your senses, not
just your eyes. Walk outside and, using
sheets of paper and coloured pencils,
make rubbings of textures and patterns
you find on different surfaces, such as
tables, brick walls, and tree trunks.
Once finished, cut out or arrange the
patterns into a collage. You can overlap
them, join them together, or even turn
them into a landscape.

SELF-REFLECTION What was it like to
explore life through your sense of touch
and capture patterns that are often
overlooked? Did you find it relaxing
or soothing to concentrate on sensory
input? Could there be areas of your life
where you could focus more on your
feelings instead of thoughts?

015

Colouring outside the lines

Try this when
you feel trapped by
your belief systems

You will need
Predesigned image to colour in,
coloured pencils or markers

10 minutes

Colour in a predesigned image, either in
a colouring book or something you have
drawn, without restricting yourself to
following any of the lines.

SELF-REFLECTION Were you able to colour
outside of the lines? Was it difficult or
easy? If it was easy, could this mean
you are ready to challenge your belief
systems? If it was challenging, might this
be a sign that you need to work on
stepping outside your comfort zone?
Consider how this makes you feel.

Testing out tools

If you are curious about which art tools feel most comfortable to use, try this exercise to discover your favourites. Learning your preferences can help you find your creative voice, liberating you from expectations of what art-making should look like and prioritizing what you want from the creative process.

Try this when
you need space from strong feelings

1 hour 40 minutes

016 **Fading or present**

You will need

Paper, watercolours, thick paintbrushes, thin paintbrushes

Use thin brushes to paint lines across a piece of paper, then do the same with thick brushes. Which one felt more comfortable for you? Why?

017 **Predictability or surprise?**

You will need

Paper, watercolours, sponges, rags, aluminium foil, old toothbrush

1 hour 40 minutes

Next, colour a piece of paper using sponges, rags, an old toothbrush, or scrunched-up aluminium foil. Do you notice a preference for a tool that you are finding more interesting than others?

018 **Painting with the body**

You will need

Paper, watercolours

Last, colour a sheet of paper using your fingers, hands, feet, or another body part.

SELF-REFLECTION When you have finished exploring each tool,
write down your reactions (physical, emotional, and rational) using
the template below.

tool	body	feelings	thoughts

Which tools did you prefer? Were you drawn towards traditional
tools like brushes, or did you find it more interesting to test out
unconventional equipment? Think about how creative tools can
give you space from the art experience, acting as a buffer between
the emotion you are seeking to express and your creation, reducing
feelings of overwhelm. Did using certain tools make you feel more
distant or more connected to your emotions?

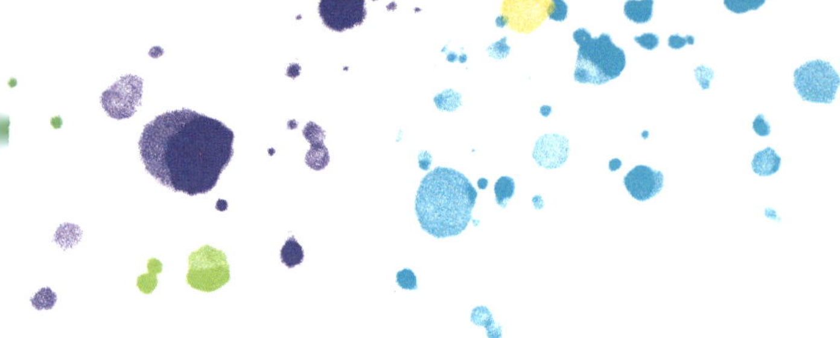

019

Blind drawing

Try this when
you want to challenge your
ideas about beauty

You will need
Paper, pencil

10 minutes

To become more expressive, try letting go of the expectation that art needs to look a certain way to be valuable or meaningful. In art therapy, this isn't true at all. Choose an object or a person to draw and, without looking at your paper, let your hand move freely while you draw, focusing only on observing the subject rather than making a perfect image.

SELF-REFLECTION How did it feel to paint something without the need to make it look perfect? Were you upset by your finished drawing? Perhaps you aren't allowing yourself to create freely because you are focused on a fixed concept of beauty or aesthetics. Where does this idea come from?

REMEMBER In art therapy, the focus is around the process and the story, not the end product.

020

Non-dominant
hand drawing

Try this when
you want to break out
of your mould

You will need
Paper, pencil

10 minutes

Create a drawing or doodle using only your non-dominant hand. Keep the focus on the creative experience rather than the result.

SELF-REFLECTION What emotions arose within you as you worked with your non-dominant hand? Did you notice a difference in how you approached the process? Could you use this exercise to stretch yourself outside your creative comfort zone?

021

Transforming mistakes

Try this when
you want to challenge
your ideas about art

You will need
Paper, pen, cup of
coffee or tea

10 minutes

Thinking outside the box and using everyday things to make art expands our creative capacity. Spill some coffee or tea onto a sheet of paper and let it dry. Try to identify symbols or figures that emerge from it, or see if you can transform the spill into a recognizable object or abstract piece of art using a pen.

SELF-REFLECTION Did you notice the creative potential? Or was it hard? Could this be a reflection of your own beliefs about your ability to create meaningful art?

022

Impossible art test

Try this when
you feel limited by rules and expectations

You will need
Paper, markers, coloured pencils, pen

10 minutes

Either on separate pieces of paper or on one piece, first draw a simple object using two markers at once. Then, just use dots or squiggles to create an image. Finally, draw without lifting your pen from the paper, switching hands every 30 seconds. You can either focus on one challenge per drawing, or try combining all of them together to create one piece. It's your choice.

SELF-REFLECTION How did it feel to create with an unconventional "rule"? Did you enjoy imposing your own guidelines? Did you discover new ways of making art? How can breaking the "rules" lead to more creativity, both in your artistic expression and personal life?

023

Rotating art

Try this when
you want to explore new perspectives

You will need
Paper, pencil, eraser, coloured pencils

20 minutes

Draw ten flowers. Turn the paper 90 degrees and draw ten more flowers, continuing until the page is full. Notice how altering the perspective of a drawing can give you a different understanding of the composition and allow for more creative possibilities.

SELF-REFLECTION Were you able to find flow due to the changing perspectives? Or did it feel disruptive? How might these shifts in perspective relate to how you navigate change in other areas of your life?

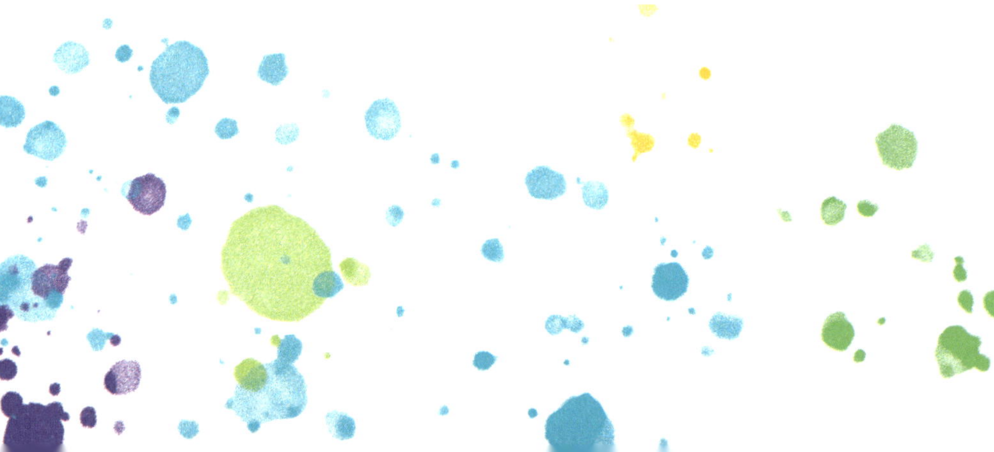

024

Messy art challenge

Try this when
you are ready to freely
express yourself

You will need
Paper, markers, watercolours or
mixed media, paintbrushes

25 minutes

Thinking that art must be orderly and
neat can limit our creativity and ability
to use it as a healing tool. Fill a piece of
paper with random colours, marks, and
shapes, making it as messy as possible.
Then, draw at least three more layers on
top, adding more colours, different-sized
scribbles, words, or symbols. Keep
drawing layers until the page is full.

SELF-REFLECTION Did you feel resistance
to making a "mess"? Why? Are there
inherited belief systems about the art
world that are influencing your creative
choices? Can letting go of neatness help
you to use art for self-healing?

025

Destructive art transformation

Try this when
you feel afraid of making mistakes

You will need
Paper, markers, paint

20 minutes

Create a simple drawing or painting, then
destroy it on purpose in some way: rip it,
cut it, crumple it, or paint over it. Observe
how you feel about your art being
"ruined". If necessary, take deep breaths
and remind yourself that this is just
colour on paper and you are expanding
your horizons about what art can be.
Once you have given yourself permission
to be uncomfortable, transform the
wrecked art into something new by using
collage, layering, or reconstructing it.
Notice how it feels to take control of the
art and make it your own again.

SELF-REFLECTION How did it feel to
"destroy" your own artwork? Did letting
go of the original image allow you to see
how much more art can be? What does
this process teach you about how art can
help you understand that it is okay for it
to be messy and ugly?

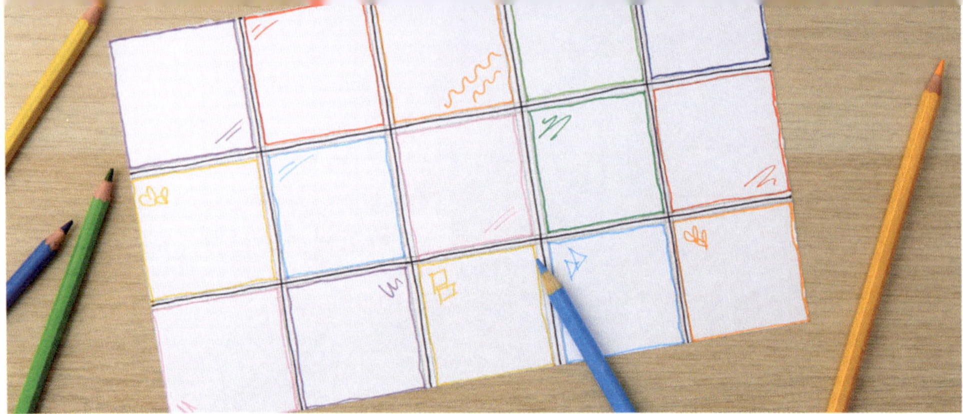

026

Nature's blueprint

Try this when
you want to calm your mind

You will need
Paper, pencil, markers,
coloured pencils

30 minutes

The repetitive rhythm of drawing patterns
can help to regulate emotions, slowing
heart rate and breathing. Go outside and
observe the natural patterns around you
- leaf veins, tree bark, rippling water,
raindrops, and so on. Sketch or trace
these on paper, then use coloured
pencils or markers to draw more until
you fill the whole page.

SELF-REFLECTION How did it feel to
recreate patterns? Was it soothing? What
repeat designs in nature stood out to
you? Why do you think they caught your
attention? Do you see any connections
between these natural patterns and
patterns in your own life?

027

Humans' blueprint

Try this when
you want to break habits
that no longer serve you

You will need
Paper, pencil, markers, coloured pencils

30 minutes

Recognizing and adapting patterns in
art can mirror personal growth, offering
insights into habitual behaviours and the
possibility of change. Walk outside and
look at the patterns found in buildings,
tiles, fences, or shadows cast by objects.
Then, choose one that interests you and
recreate it, giving it your own twist -
altering colours, breaking symmetry, or
blending different patterns together.

SELF-REFLECTION Why do you think
particular patterns caught your attention?
Did you feel the need to keep the pattern
structured, or did you enjoy changing it?
What does that say about your approach
to control and flexibility?

028

Geometric zoo

Try this when
you want to explore how
you approach challenges

You will need
Paper, pencil, eraser,
markers, coloured pencils

30 minutes

Draw simple geometric shapes to create animals, including a lion, giraffe, monkey, bear, elephant, and wolf, then colour them in.

SELF-REFLECTION How did you find the process of designing these abstract creations? Did it feel challenging or interesting? Could this relate to how you approach complex challenges in life?

029

Parallel painting

Try this when
you want to regain balance

You will need
Two pieces of paper,
coloured pencils, timer

20+ minutes

Set a timer for 5 minutes, and use fast, bold marks and dark colours to create an expressive and chaotic composition. For another 5 minutes, on a second piece of paper, focus on soft, organized lines with light colours to create a calm image. Switch between the two for another round of 5 minutes each.

SELF-REFLECTION How did it feel to shift between these two compositions? Did you find yourself resisting one approach? How do you experience the shift between chaos and calm in daily life?

030

Unique artistic voice

Try this when
you are ready to welcome
your new artistic self

You will need
Materials you enjoyed
during this chapter, paper

30+ minutes

Recognize which artistic choices you gravitated towards the most in this chapter. Create an art piece using all the techniques, materials, colours, and tools that you enjoyed and felt the most comfortable with. Repeat this exercise as many times as you like.

SELF-REFLECTION Why do you think your choices felt comfortable or enjoyable? Were there any patterns or tendencies you noticed across multiple attempts? Were there surprises? How might these inform your future creative explorations?

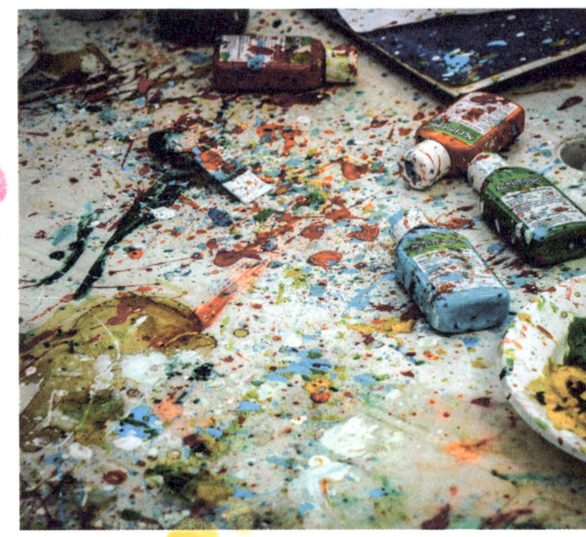

Letting go of perfection

Striving for perfection may seem like a noble pursuit, but it can lead to failure. When we create art, the focus should be on the process rather than achieving a beautiful end result. These exercises aim to help you detach from the notion that art (and you) must be perfect in order to be worthwhile.

031

The ugliest creation

Try this when
you are ready to
embrace your flaws

You will need
Any art materials
you have at hand

10 minutes

Create the ugliest piece you can. Deliberately lay
down wonky lines, use colours you find unpleasant,
and exaggerate flaws. When you've finished, reflect
on how it feels to look at it. Is it grotesque? Good.
That means you can't possibly make anything that's
worse. And if it isn't, then perhaps you shouldn't
worry so much about imperfection.

SELF-REFLECTION Were you able to create something
unpleasant without being too harsh on yourself?
Does this reveal anything about how perfectionism
affects you? What could this say about accepting
your own flaws and still seeing your true value?

032

Intuition mapping

Try this when
you feel disconnected
from yourself

You will need
Paper, pencil, coloured
pencils, markers

10 minutes

Close your eyes and try to tune in to your intuition
and inner wisdom. Is your heart speaking to you?
Do you have a gut feeling? Draw a stick figure, then
using coloured pencils or markers, mark where your
body is expressing this.

SELF-REFLECTION Were you able to connect with
your body's expression of intuition? Are there any
particular parts of your body that speak to you?
How can connecting with these parts of yourself
allow you to identify your needs and create space
for self-acceptance?

Your inner critic and inner wisdom

The inner critic is the voice inside our heads that highlights our fears and limitations. It often stems from past negative experiences or societal expectations. Recognizing your inner critic can help you challenge it, giving you space to become more self-accepting. Your inner wisdom, or the intuitive self, draws on the knowledge you have gained from your body's experiences, guiding you towards your natural insights, strengths, and desires.

Try this when
you feel overpowered by self-criticism

60 minutes

033 Meeting your inner critic

You will need

Paper, pencil, coloured pencils, markers

Draw a figure that represents your inner critic. This can take any shape you like, and can be as detailed or as abstract as you wish. Pretend it is a character from a film. When it's complete, write the following around the outside of it: their name, likes and dislikes, and what makes them stronger or weaker.

034 Connecting with your inner critic

You will need

Paper, pencil, coloured pencils, markers

Now, draw some thought bubbles on the same piece of paper as the last exercise. Then, write some of the phrases you constantly hear your inner critic say to you inside them. For example: "Why would you do that?" "What will people think?" "That's not good enough", and so on.

035 **Meeting your inner wisdom**

You will need

Paper, pencil, coloured
pencils, markers

Next, draw a figure that represents your
inner wisdom. Again, this can take any
form and include a lot of detail or be
fairly abstract. Pretend this is a film
character and build a profile around it,
writing down their name, likes and
dislikes, and their superpowers and
weaknesses.

036 **Connecting with your
inner wisdom**

You will need

Paper, pencil, coloured
pencils, markers

Last, draw a heart on another piece
of paper and write down anything
that helps you to identify your inner
wisdom. Some examples include: "my
gut feeling tells me", "having a clear
mind", "a sense of deep knowing", and
"a feeling of flow".

SELF-REFLECTION Were you able to laugh about the characters you
created, or did they feel threatening? This could be a reflection of
how hard you are on yourself. Were you able to see these parts of
yourself in a different light and embrace them? Or did they feel like
something you want to reject? Were you able to connect with your
inner wisdom? Could you start listening more to your inner wisdom
instead of the perfectionist voice of your inner critic?

037

The one-line drawing

Try this when
you need to break through
a creative block

You will need
Paper, pencil, coloured pencils,
markers

10 minutes

Choose one or two objects around you,
such as a plant, mug, or your hand, and
draw them without lifting your pencil
or marker from the page. Let the lines
connect in unexpected ways and avoid
erasing or correcting any "mistakes".
Use different colours to layer over
the drawing.

SELF-REFLECTION What emotions arose
while you were drawing without stopping
or correcting? Was there something that
surprised you about your result? How can
you connect your creative experience
with your feelings towards perfectionism?

038

The permission letter

Try this when
you feel lost on your artistic journey

You will need
Paper, pencil, pen

20 minutes

Sit down, and, if it is comfortable to do
so, close your eyes and imagine yourself
as a teenager. Notice where you are,
what you look like, and the clothes and
accessories you are wearing. Imagine
having a conversation with that version
of yourself, asking what kind of artist they
want to be. Thank this version of yourself
for their wisdom. When you're ready,
open your eyes and note what comes to
mind. Write a letter to your teenage self,
encouraging them to create art in the
way they once dreamed. Remind them
that you are proud of them and fully
support their creativity. Put this letter in
a safe place for you to read when you
are feeling creatively disengaged.

SELF-REFLECTION Was it easy or difficult
to connect with your inner adolescent?
Is the art that came up during your
visualization different from what you
already make? Can this insight serve as
inspiration to find a new way to create
art today?

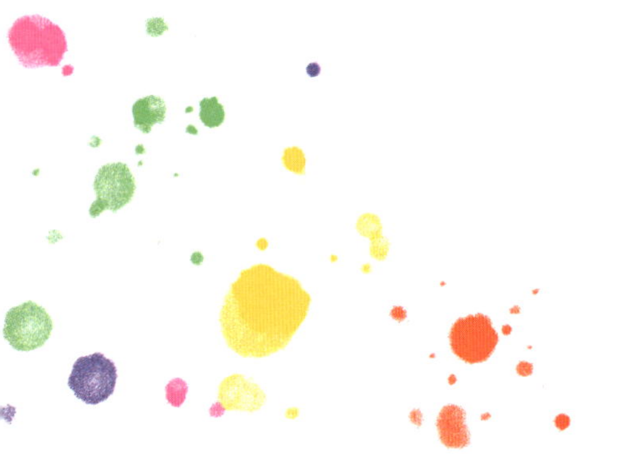

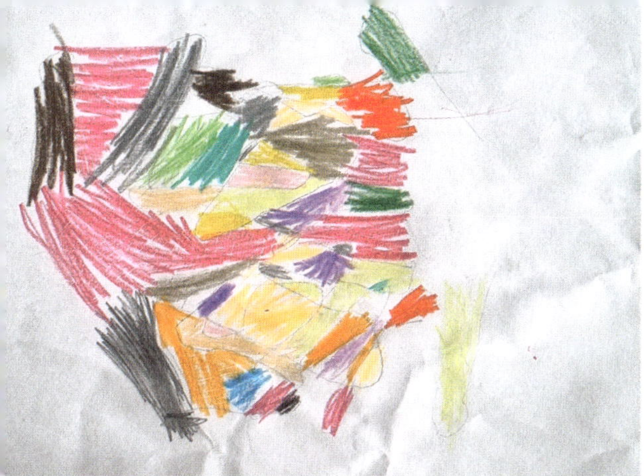

039

There is beauty in imperfection

Try this when
you are being too hard
on yourself

You will need
Paper, pencil, coloured
pencils

30 minutes

Scrunch a piece of paper into a ball, then open it up
and try to smooth it back into its original form. You
will notice that the paper is covered in wrinkled lines.
Highlight all these lines with a pencil. When you have
finished, use coloured pencils to colour in as many of
the blank spaces in between the lines as you like. Try
to see the beauty that has emerged out of something
"broken".

SELF-REFLECTION Was this a difficult process for you,
or did you enjoy it? What emotions or thoughts came
up for you? Could this mean you are able to find
beauty in imperfection?

040

Art is everywhere

Try this when
you feel uninspired

You will need
Phone camera

30 minutes

Walk around your neighbourhood and look for
"accidental art" that hasn't been created deliberately,
but you find beautiful or interesting. It could be a pile
of leaves, pipes that look like faces, or layers of old
posters on a billboard. Document these by taking
photos on your phone, then reflect on how art can be
created without intent or skill and still be captivating.

SELF-REFLECTION Did you find any accidental art in
your environment? Could this mean that art isn't only
about talent, as it can be created unintentionally?

041

Broken art

Try this when
you question your worth

You will need
Paper, pencil, markers,
coloured pencils

30 minutes

While walking outside, look for cracks in the pavement and document them by drawing them on a piece of paper. Then use a marker to outline any shapes you find hidden in these cracks. Maybe they turn into a face, a dragon, or a landscape? You can colour them in if you want.

SELF-REFLECTION Notice how stopping to observe the brokenness of the world can inspire awe and maybe even help you find magic. What does this process say about your ability to discover value in overlooked things (or parts of yourself)?

042

Letting go of inadequacy

Try this when
you want to release
self-doubt

You will need
Paper, watercolours,
paintbrushes, water

20 minutes

Think of a situation that made you feel like you weren't "good enough". Using watercolours, identify three colours that represent that feeling for you, then fill a piece of paper with them. Let the paper dry, then slowly tear it into smaller pieces, giving yourself permission to let go of these feelings. You may discard the pieces or save them for a future artwork.

SELF-REFLECTION Was breaking something in a contained manner liberating for you? Were you able to let go of those feelings, or do you still have a lingering sense of inadequacy? Are you judging yourself more harshly than you would judge someone else?

REMEMBER There are no right or wrong answers. There is no need to feel guilty if you don't perceive a difference. All the exercises are about developing self-awareness.

043

There's beauty in broken pieces

Try this when
you feel closed off to
new perspectives

You will need
Two pieces of paper,
watercolours, paintbrushes,
water, scissors, tape or glue

30 minutes

Fill two pages with colours that you don't like or that you feel don't combine well together. If you notice this is making you uncomfortable, take a deep breath and, while slowly exhaling, tell yourself that this kind of discomfort is okay. When you are finished, cut both papers into smaller pieces and use them to make a mosaic.

SELF-REFLECTION Was there a transformation in your opinion about the colour combinations, or did it stay the same? Did changing the form help to reframe your ideas or opinions? Does this mean that there's value in things that are far from perfect? Could it be that our own brokenness can also be cherished?

044

The ruined painting

Try this when
you are ready to let go
of perfectionism

You will need
Paper, watercolours,
paintbrushes, water,
markers, pencils

15 minutes

Using watercolours, create a small painting with soft washes of colour. Let the painting dry, then use a marker to "ruin" it by drawing bold lines, doodles, or scribbles on top. Notice any resistance that arises and breathe deeply through it, just as you did in the previous exercise. Try to transform the "ruined" parts by incorporating them into the artwork.

SELF-REFLECTION What was your initial reaction to "ruining" your painting? How did it feel to transform the imperfections into something new? In what ways might you be able to embrace imperfections in other areas of your life?

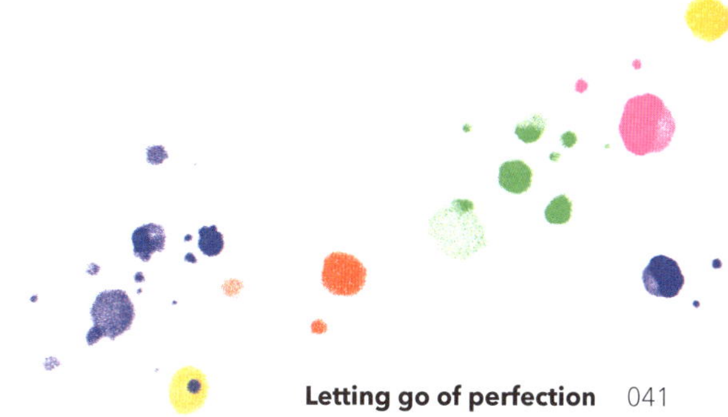

045

My success timeline

Try this when
you feel overwhelmed
by challenges

You will need
Paper, ruler, markers, pen

15 minutes

Draw a straight line across the whole page with a ruler, then use this to create a timeline representing yourself. Draw your younger self at one end and the current version of you at the opposite end. Think of five challenging times that you overcame in your life, and put them on the timeline. At each point, write down things that helped you through that episode.

SELF-REFLECTION Were you able to identify events you have overcome? How did it feel to review them? Were you able to recognize your own coping skills?

046

My failure timeline

Try this when
you want to reflect on your
personal growth

You will need
Paper, ruler, markers, pen

15 minutes

Draw a straight line across the page and use it as a timeline to represent yourself. Again, draw your younger self at one end and the current version of you at the other. Think of five times where you failed and put them on the timeline. For each, write down how you coped with the mistakes and what lessons you learned. Give yourself recognition for having survived those difficult times, and think about how you grew wiser from those moments.

SELF-REFLECTION Were you able to name previous mistakes? How did it feel to see them in front of you? Were you able to hold yourself kindly?

047

Scribble transformation

Try this when
you feel doubtful about
your ability to cope

You will need
Paper, pencil

15 minutes

With your eyes closed, draw a random scribble. Open your eyes and transform it into a creature, character, or object by adding as many details as you wish.

SELF-REFLECTION Were you able to create something out of randomness? Did you find yourself wanting to "correct" your scribble? What does this show you about your own adaptability?

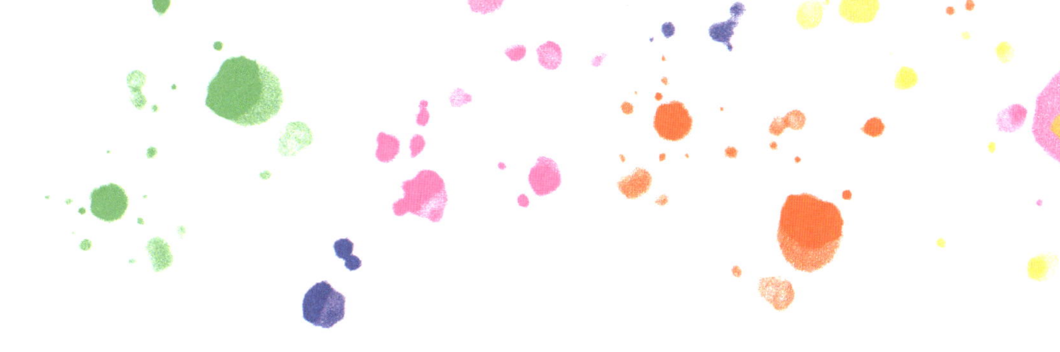

048

Letting go of control part 1

Try this when
you want to get comfortable
with discomfort

You will need
Paper, marker, coloured pencils

15 minutes

Using a marker and your non-dominant
hand, trace the outline of your dominant
hand onto paper. Then, still with your
non-dominant hand, use different colours
to colour it in. Notice how it feels to
create in this new way.

SELF-REFLECTION Was this an easy or
challenging process? Did you find
yourself wanting to go back to your
dominant hand? Could this be a mini
reflection of how difficult it can be to let
go of control?

REMEMBER It's okay not to be in complete
control all the time.

049

Letting go of control part 2

Try this when
you want to build your
frustration tolerance

You will need
Paper, pencil, eraser

15 minutes

Draw a self-portrait or a simple object
using your non-dominant hand. Notice
how the process feels, and use your eraser
if necessary. If it's too uncomfortable,
remember to breathe and remind yourself
that this is helping you get comfortable
with trying out new things.

SELF-REFLECTION Were you frustrated that
your art didn't look as you expected?
Were you able to step away and breathe
when you felt uncomfortable, and return
to finish? How much erasing were you
doing? Are you fixating too much on how
it looks instead of celebrating that you are
taking a risk and trying new things?

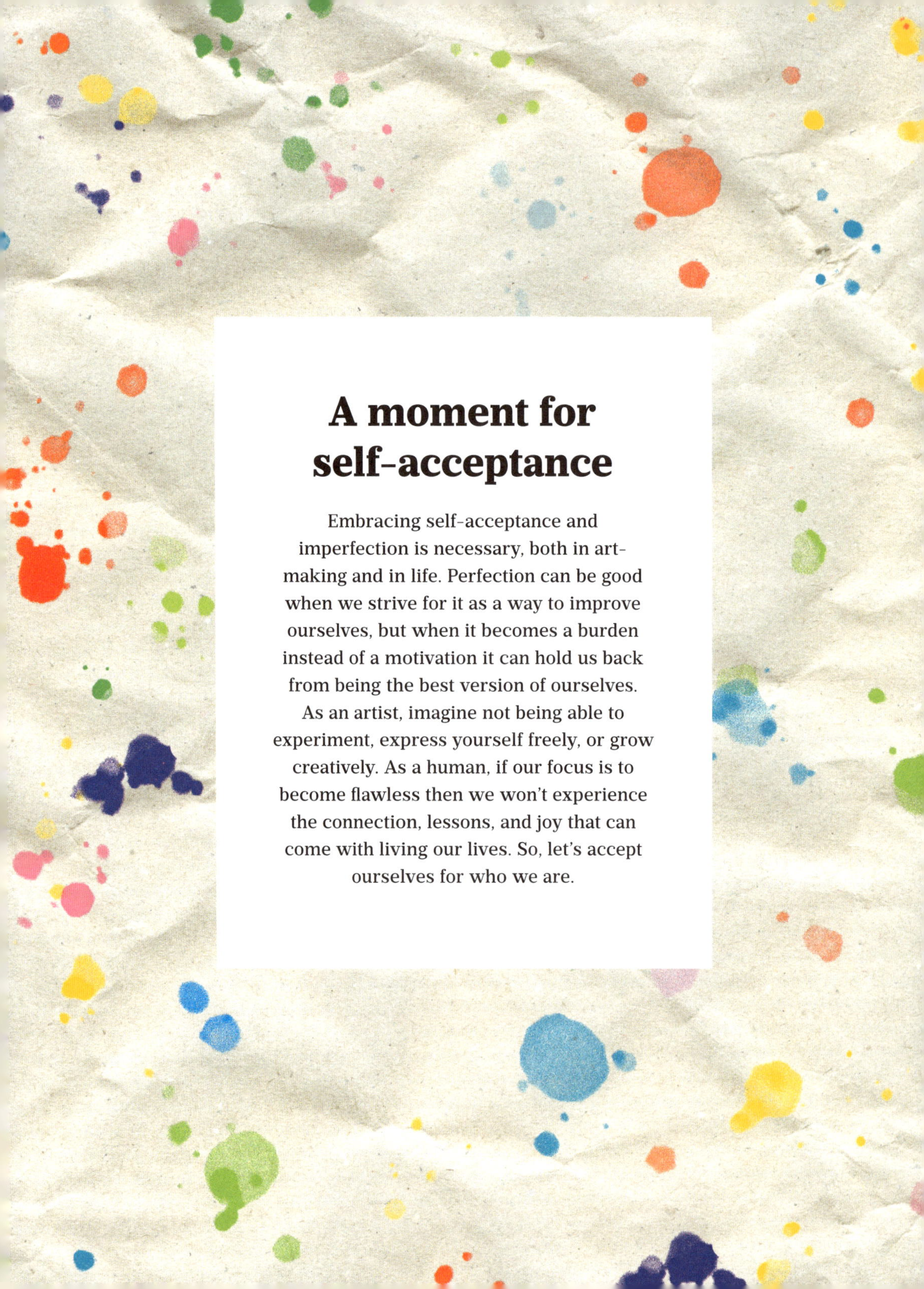

A moment for self-acceptance

Embracing self-acceptance and imperfection is necessary, both in art-making and in life. Perfection can be good when we strive for it as a way to improve ourselves, but when it becomes a burden instead of a motivation it can hold us back from being the best version of ourselves. As an artist, imagine not being able to experiment, express yourself freely, or grow creatively. As a human, if our focus is to become flawless then we won't experience the connection, lessons, and joy that can come with living our lives. So, let's accept ourselves for who we are.

050

Correcting mistakes

Try this when
you are struggling to cope

You will need
Paper, coloured pencils,
markers

20 minutes

By creating an imaginary problem and solving it, we can show that we can adapt during times of trouble. Using just coloured pencils, draw a person who is experiencing car trouble. When you've finished, use markers to draw potential solutions to the problem.

SELF-REFLECTION Were you able to assist the figure in the drawing? Did you notice how your creativity kicked in when a challenge was presented? Can you trust your intuition to fix things when necessary?

051

The perfect vs the real me

Try this when
you feel overwhelmed by
the pressure to be perfect

You will need
Paper, coloured pencils,
markers

20 minutes

Building awareness around our own expectations of perfection is the first step towards combating it. Divide a piece of paper into two sections. On one side, draw a representation of yourself that shows a "perfect" version of you – the one you feel pressured to be. On the other side, depict your authentic self, including both your strengths and imperfections.

SELF-REFLECTION What expectations shape your "perfect" self? How do you feel when comparing both sides? What aspects of your real self do you want to embrace more?

052

Tightrope perfection

Try this when
you want to challenge
your perfectionism

You will need
Paper, pencils, markers

20 minutes

Draw a tightrope stretching across the whole page. On one side, illustrate or write the rewards of striving for perfection, and on the other, show the costs or burdens. Finally, draw yourself walking this tightrope, representing your personal experience with perfectionism – for example, are you confidently striding, or wobbling with the strain?

SELF-REFLECTION What drives you to stay on this tightrope? Is the effort to maintain balance worth the cost? How could you make space for more flexibility?

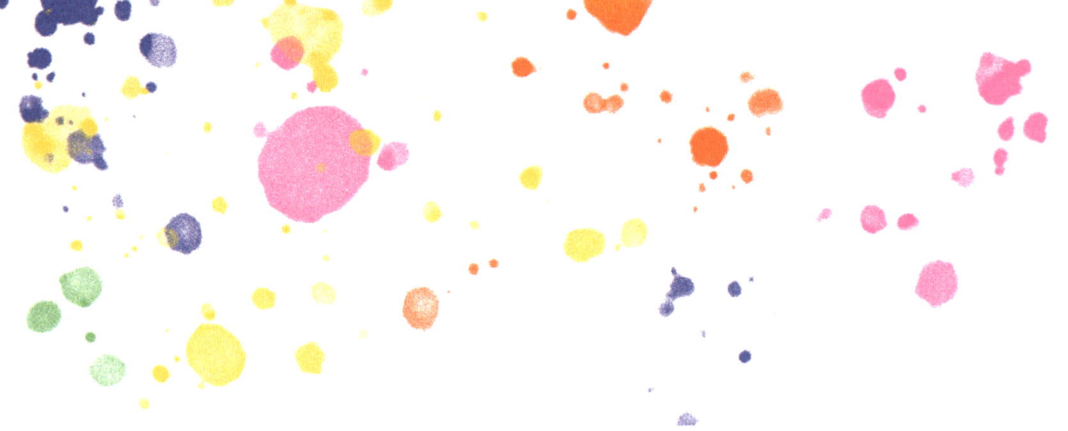

053

Erased lines

Try this when
you want to challenge
your inner critic

You will need
Paper, pencil, eraser,
markers, timer

30 minutes

First, use a pencil to draw a detailed image of a
floral bouquet, then spend 5 minutes erasing and
redrawing parts to make it "better". Pause and reflect
on how it feels to keep adjusting the drawing. When
you feel it's complete, use markers to go over the
lines boldly, accepting them as they are.

SELF-REFLECTION How did it feel to keep changing
your drawing? At what point were you satisfied - if
ever? What would happen if you let go of the need
for constant revision?

054

Upside-down
self-portrait

Try this when
you want to practise
self-acceptance

You will need
Pencil, eraser, markers,
coloured pencils, phone
camera or mirror

10 minutes

Draw the outline of a face and neck, then flip the
paper upside down. Then, looking at yourself in a
mirror or on your phone's camera, try to draw your
facial features while keeping the paper upside down.
It might feel tricky, but let go of perfection and just
focus on observing. Finally, place the drawing
right-side up and see how it turned out.

SELF-REFLECTION Were you able to create while
working upside down? Are you okay with how the
drawing looked or not? If you are not content with
your creation, could this reaction be more about your
focus on how you think things should be instead of
accepting things as they are?

055

Trophy shelf part 1

Try this when
you want to celebrate
your achievements

You will need
Paper, pencil, markers,
coloured pencils

20 minutes

Draw a shelf and fill it with symbolic or
literal trophies, awards, or diplomas
that represent your past successes or
achievements that you are proud of.

SELF-REFLECTION Do you tend to measure
your self-worth based on achievements?
Was it easy to name all of your awards?

056

Trophy shelf part 2

Try this when
you want to celebrate
personal growth

You will need
Paper, pencil, markers,
coloured pencils

20 minutes

Draw a shelf, then fill it with awards
for personal moments of growth,
connection, or happiness that weren't
just about achievement. For example,
think of a time you supported a friend
through a difficult period, improved your
relationship with your partner, family,
or children, or a time when you helped
someone in need.

SELF-REFLECTION Think of the shelf you
drew in the previous exercise. Which
one feels more fulfilling to you? What
non-achievement-based values do you
want to honour more?

057

Permission slip part 1

Try this when
you are ready to
accept your flaws

You will need
Paper, pencil, markers,
coloured pencils

20 minutes

Design a "permission slip" for yourself, allowing for flaws in an area of your life where you feel the most pressure to be perfect. Decorate it with colours, images, or affirmations that remind you imperfection is part of growth. Make copies and keep them somewhere handy for whenever you need them.

SELF-REFLECTION In what area of your life do you struggle to accept imperfection? How does it feel to grant yourself permission?

058

Permission slip part 2

Try this when
you want to listen to
your inner voice

You will need
Paper, pencil, markers,
coloured pencils

20 minutes

The focus of this exercise is to connect with one of your inner strengths – your intuition. Design a second "permission slip", this time allowing yourself to use your intuitive voice and be more creative. Utilize colours, images, or affirmations that remind you that your inner voice matters.

SELF-REFLECTION In what area of life do you struggle to welcome your intuitive voice? How does it feel to give yourself permission to follow your gut instinct instead of your rational mind?

059

Stained creature

Try this when
you need to break out of
your comfort zone

You will need
Napkin, pen

15 minutes

After finishing a meal, look at your used napkin and observe the stains left behind. Instead of seeing them as messy or imperfect, look for shapes, patterns, or hidden entities within them. Use a pen to outline and transform the stain into a creature, adding as many details as you wish to bring it to life.

SELF-REFLECTION How did it feel to create something from a stain rather than a planned design? Did you notice any resistance to working with something "imperfect"? How might embracing unexpected outcomes lead to new possibilities in your life?

Mask of hidden truths

Try this when

you want to see your flaws in a new light

You will need

Old boxes, recyclable materials (e.g. plastic caps or egg cartons), tape, scissors

30 minutes

Use old boxes and recyclable materials to create a mask that represents how you present yourself to the world. When your mask is finished, use colours, textures, or words on the inside to symbolize the emotions or aspects of yourself that are often hidden. You might wish to scratch the cardboard, place tape unevenly, or take advantage of the textures of the recycled materials.

SELF-REFLECTION How did you find the experience of creating art with what could be considered rubbish? Is there a possibility that even old or unusable things can be repurposed into something meaningful? Could this apply to your own perceived weaknesses? How might what you see as a limitation become a hidden strength?

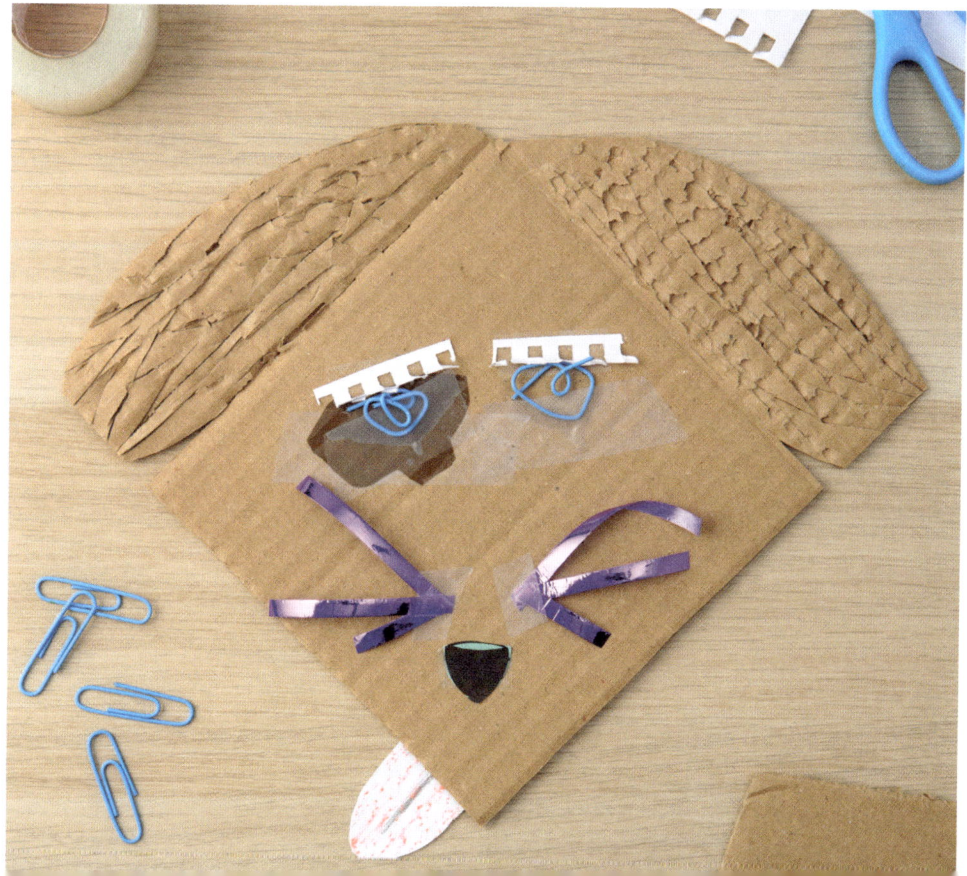

Finding yourself through creativity

The creative process offers a powerful path to self-discovery. When you create art, you tap into thoughts and emotions that may be difficult to access through language. Art allows you to externalize what's inside, offering new perspectives on your experiences and beliefs. By embracing the creative process without judgement, you can open the door to deeper self-awareness and personal growth.

061

Collage as a path for self-discovery

Try this when
you feel unsure of
who you are

You will need
Paper, magazine or
printouts of images,
scissors, glue, markers,
coloured pencils or
mixed media

25 minutes

Self-portraits offer a mirror of our inner world, helping us see ourselves with clarity and compassion. Gather your materials and take a moment to sit with the age-old question, "who am I?" Then use the materials to create an image that represents you. You can include the whole of your personality or just parts you are proud of, things you like, and the roles you play in your life. You can do this through symbols as well as images. Take a moment to examine your finished piece.

SELF-REFLECTION What aspects of your self-portrait stand out to you the most? Do these define you? If not, what could you add to represent you better? If you want, you can add them after finishing this reflective moment.

062

Who am I?

Try this when
you want to get to
know yourself better

You will need
Paper, watercolours
or mixed media

25 minutes

Think about the colours that represent different parts of your personality – the roles you play, your strengths, and your values (see pp.10–13 for inspiration). Once you've chosen a colour code for the different aspects of yourself, use those colours to create an abstract representation of who you are. Let your artwork dry, then take time to reflect on your creation.

SELF-REFLECTION What colours stand out to you the most? Do you think those colours represent the most important parts of you? Or did they surprise you? Could this be a reflection of how others see you?

063

Blind self-portrait

Try this when
you want to connect with
your creative self

You will need
Phone camera, paper, marker

10 minutes

Open your phone camera to see your
reflection. Without looking away, begin
drawing your face on a piece of paper,
keeping your eyes on your reflection
the entire time. Do not lift your hand
while drawing but let your lines flow
continuously. Take a moment to look
at your creation once complete.

SELF-REFLECTION How did it feel to draw
without looking? Were you focused on
the experience, or were you worried
about how the portrait would turn out?
Was it hard to let go during the creative
process or was it liberating? What
could this process tell you about your
creative self?

REMEMBER This exercise can be intense,
as looking at yourself for a prolonged
period is something we are not used to.
Be patient and kind with yourself.

064

The many sides of me

Try this when
you are ready to embrace your
whole self

You will need
Paper, magazine cutouts or image
printouts, scissors, glue, markers,
coloured pencils or mixed media

30 minutes

We hold many different ways of existing
within ourselves, so let's acknowledge
them all. Gather your materials and
create a collage that represents the
different roles or identities you hold in
life, such as daughter/son, friend, partner,
caregiver, artist, worker, dreamer, thinker,
and so on. Use both images and words
to represent them.

SELF-REFLECTION Which identities feel
strongest to you? Are there parts of
yourself you wish you had more space
for? What would a more balanced
version of these identities look like?

065

My inner landscape part 1

Try this when
you want to explore your inner world

You will need
Paper, coloured pencils

25 minutes

Take some time to connect with yourself and think about how you see your inner and outer worlds. Spark your imagination by thinking of your inner world as a landscape. What would best represent you? Are you a stormy sea, a vast desert, or a lush forest? Draw what comes to mind.

SELF-REFLECTION What does landscape reveal about how you see yourself? How does it compare to the way you view your outer world? What might it tell you about your awareness of your feelings and your surroundings?

066

My inner landscape part 2

Try this when
you want to expand your vision of yourself

You will need
Paper, paint, sponges, toothbrush, aluminium foil

25 minutes

Connect with your body by recreating the same landscape as in the previous exercise, but this time use your hands or an unusual artistic tool, like a toothbrush or sponge, instead of a paintbrush.

SELF-REFLECTION Was the experience of creating with your hands and using alternative materials more challenging or enjoyable? Were your thoughts racing when creating this image, or was your mind quiet and focused on the process? Could experimenting with different creative styles be revealing hidden aspects of yourself or unlocking new ways of understanding your emotions?

067

My name, my identity

Try this when
you feel disconnected

You will need
Paper, pen, coloured pencils

20 minutes

Exploring your name through art can uncover deep connections to identity. First write your name in large letters, then fill the spaces inside and around the letters with words that describe who you are. Add colours to words that you feel define you the most.

SELF-REFLECTION How does your name shape your identity? Does your name have a specific story tied to it that has influenced the way you are? What words did you decide to highlight? Are you proud of them?

068

The tree of growth

Try this when
you want to nurture
your strengths

You will need
Paper, pencil, pen, eraser,
watercolours, paintbrushes

20 minutes

Draw a tree with roots, a trunk, and branches. Next, write the names of people who support you on the roots, list your personal strengths along the trunk, and write challenges or areas where you would like to grow on the branches. Decorate your tree with colours that feel meaningful to you.

SELF-REFLECTION How can visualizing yourself as a tree help shift your perspective to a growth mindset? How can you use your strengths to overcome any challenges you're facing? What small steps can you take to nurture your own growth?

069

Inside vs outside self

Try this when
you feel like you can't
be yourself

You will need
Paper, pencil, markers,
coloured pencils

20 minutes

We all have a public persona and a private self. Exploring both can reveal how aligned they are, which can be key to maintaining a balanced and healthy mindset. Fold a sheet of paper in half, as if you were going to create a greeting card. On the outside, draw how you think others perceive you, then inside draw how you see yourself.

SELF-REFLECTION Are there differences between the two sides? Why? Which side felt easier to create? How would it feel to bring more of your inner self into the outside world?

070

My mask

Try this when
you want to be
more authentic

You will need
Paper plate, markers,
coloured pencils

15 minutes

Create a mask using a paper plate. Decorate the front of the mask with symbols or words that represent the version of yourself that you show to the world. Then, on the back, draw or write about the parts of yourself that people don't always see.

SELF-REFLECTION What aspects of yourself do you feel comfortable showing? What parts of yourself do you hide? Why? How would it feel to reveal more of your authentic self to others?

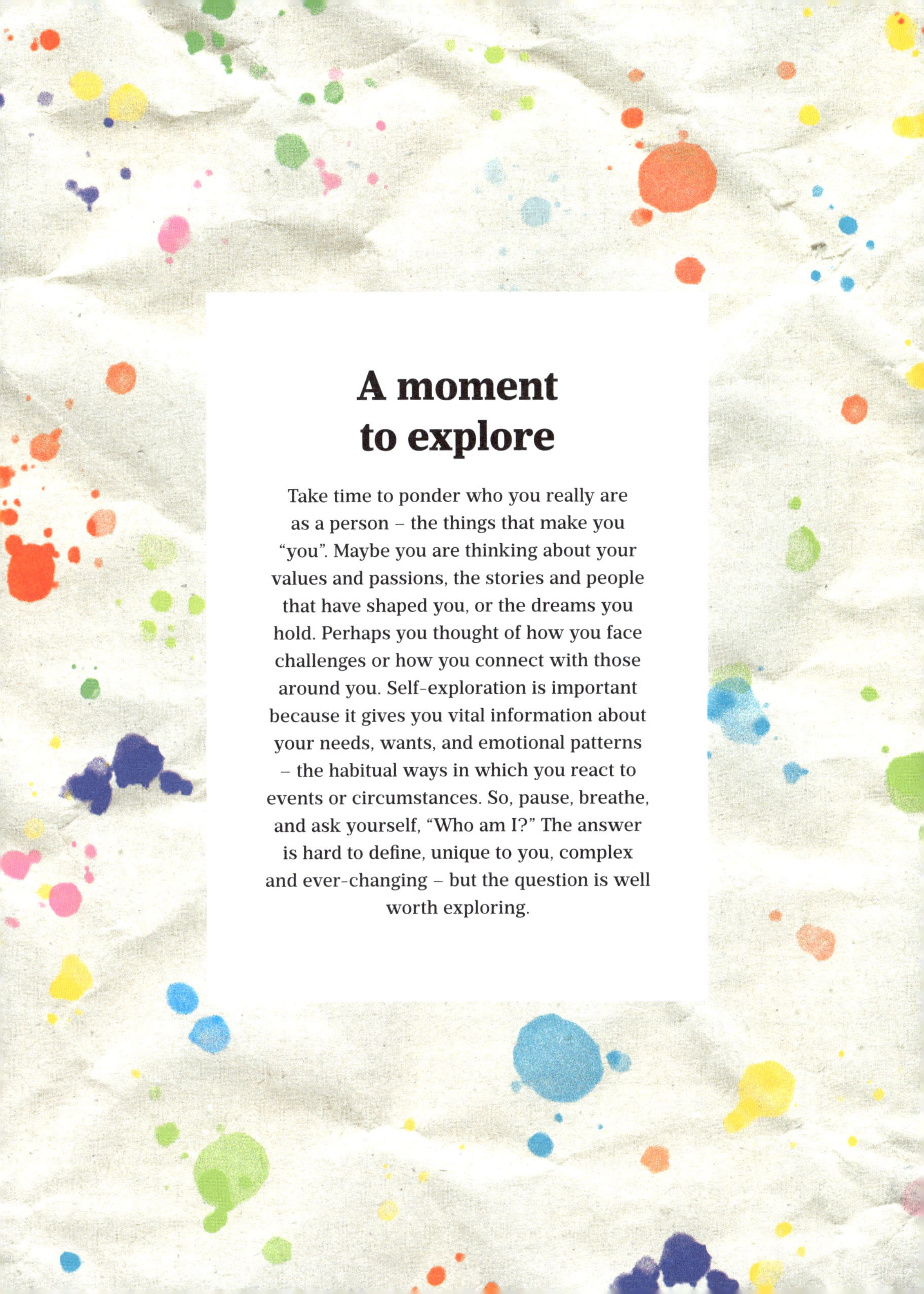

A moment to explore

Take time to ponder who you really are as a person – the things that make you "you". Maybe you are thinking about your values and passions, the stories and people that have shaped you, or the dreams you hold. Perhaps you thought of how you face challenges or how you connect with those around you. Self-exploration is important because it gives you vital information about your needs, wants, and emotional patterns – the habitual ways in which you react to events or circumstances. So, pause, breathe, and ask yourself, "Who am I?" The answer is hard to define, unique to you, complex and ever-changing – but the question is well worth exploring.

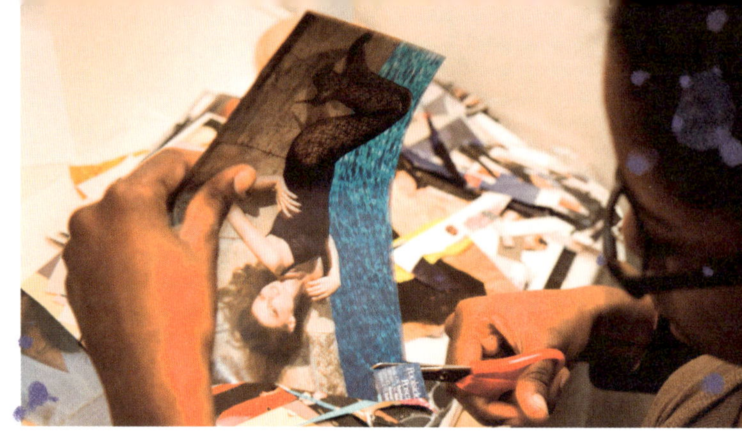

071

Future visions part 1

Try this when
you want to gain direction and purpose

You will need
Paper, magazine or image printouts, scissors, glue, markers, coloured pencils

25 minutes

Draw or create a collage representing your future aspirations. Include themes such as work, personal relationships, and significant purchases you wish to make. Include any colours, words, or images that align with your hopes and expectations. Allow yourself to dream big.

SELF-REFLECTION Was it difficult to put your dreams on paper? Did you let yourself dream big? If not, could this reflect a fear of not being able to achieve your dreams?

072

Future visions part 2

Try this when
you want to connect with your future self

You will need
Paper, magazine or image printouts, scissors, glue, markers, coloured pencils

25 minutes

Draw or create a collage representing who you want to become in the future in order to achieve your aspirations. Consider including areas where you see potential for personal growth – perhaps you need to work on emotional intelligence, improving creativity, or increasing self-confidence, for example. Use colour and images to represent different parts of yourself.

SELF-REFLECTION How does this vision align with who you are today? What small steps can you take to move towards this future self? What self-limiting beliefs do you need to let go of?

073

Postcard from the past

Try this when
you want to celebrate yourself

You will need
Paper, markers, coloured pencils,
mixed media

15 minutes

Create a postcard from the perspective
of a past version of yourself, or from your
inner child or adolescent. Decorate the
front of the postcard, perhaps trying to
recreate a piece of art from that era.
On the back, write a short note to your
present self, offering love and celebration
for all the things you have accomplished
since then.

SELF-REFLECTION Is your past self proud
of what you have become? Or are there
still things that are pending?

REMEMBER You can always start anew
every day!

074

Postcard from the future

Try this when
you need to break free from
self-limiting beliefs

You will need
Paper, markers, coloured pencils,
mixed media

15 minutes

Imagine yourself transported to the
future, where you are living out a dream
you deeply desire. Create a postcard
from this future realm, depicting what
you see, feel, or experience. On the back,
write a short note to your present self,
offering encouragement or advice from
your future self.

SELF-REFLECTION Do you allow yourself to
dream big or do you limit yourself? If you
are limiting yourself, what is getting in
the way? What do you need in order to
pursue a truly fulfilling life?

Intentions

If you want to be more future-orientated while maintaining a balanced mindset, start using intentions. These focus on how you want to be or feel, rather than what you aim to achieve. Unlike goals, which are typically future-focused and outcome-driven, intentions anchor you in the present moment, influencing your mindset, actions, and energy. Setting an intention involves identifying what you wish to experience in daily life, so that every step becomes part of the journey, not just a means to an end.

Try this when
you want to feel grounded and clear

1 hour 10 minutes

075 My word for the week

You will need
Pen, marker, sticky notes

15 minutes

Is there a feeling that you want to manifest in your life this week? Start by choosing a word that defines this - for example, "calm". This word will be your intention. Write it in big, bold letters on a sticky note, and place it somewhere you'll see often. When you feel overwhelmed, think of that word and question, "will this decision help me feel (intention)?"

076 Colour mapping the intentions

You will need
Paper, watercolours, paintbrushes

25 minutes

Next, select colours that represent different aspects of your intention. For example, if your intention is calmness, you might use blue for slowing down, yellow for self-compassion, and green for flexibility. Create an abstract piece by blending the colours together, letting them overlap and flow, symbolizing how your intention will naturally take shape in your life.

077 **Journey of intentions**

You will need

Paper, pencil, markers, coloured pencils

15+ minutes

Now, draw a path, river, or staircase to represent your journey of living with intention. At the start, write where you feel you are right now, and at the opposite end, where you would like to be. Add symbols, colours, or words along the path to represent small steps you'd like to take towards your intention.

078 **Affirmation card**

You will need

Index cards or thick paper, markers, watercolours, paintbrushes

15 minutes

Last, on index cards or thick paper, create affirmation cards by writing short, present-tense statements that clarify your intention; for example, "I am calm and in control". Decorate them with colours, doodles, or symbols that reinforce the feel of the intention.

SELF-REFLECTION Why did you choose that particular word for the week as an intention? Was it out of necessity to break old patterns or hope for a better future? Think about the colours you chose. How does this colour combination reflect your intention? How can you bring these colours into your life as reminders of your intention? What obstacles might arise on your journey, and how can you navigate them? Could keeping these colours and words visible as a daily reminder help?

079

Higher intentions

Try this when
you're in need of direction
and purpose

You will need
Paper, markers, coloured
pencils

15 minutes

Set an intention for the month. It could be the same
as the one you chose for the week, or it can be
something different. Write it in big, bold letters on
a large piece of paper, then decorate around it with
colours and symbols to highlight its importance.

SELF-REFLECTION How do the colours and patterns
represent your intention? Was it harder or easier
to find a long-term intention than the weekly one?
Could a part of you be afraid to fail and not
accomplish the intention?

080

Word weave

Try this when
you want to make your
goals feel more tangible

You will need
Paper, pen, markers

25 minutes

On a sheet of paper, write or place cut-out words
and phrases that represent how you want to show
up in your life (see pp.10–13 for inspiration). Create
a considered composition, enlarging or arranging
words in different directions, using colour and design
to emphasize the most important ones.

SELF-REFLECTION Which words stood out to you the
most? How do these words align with the life you
want to create? What small actions can help you
embody these intentions?

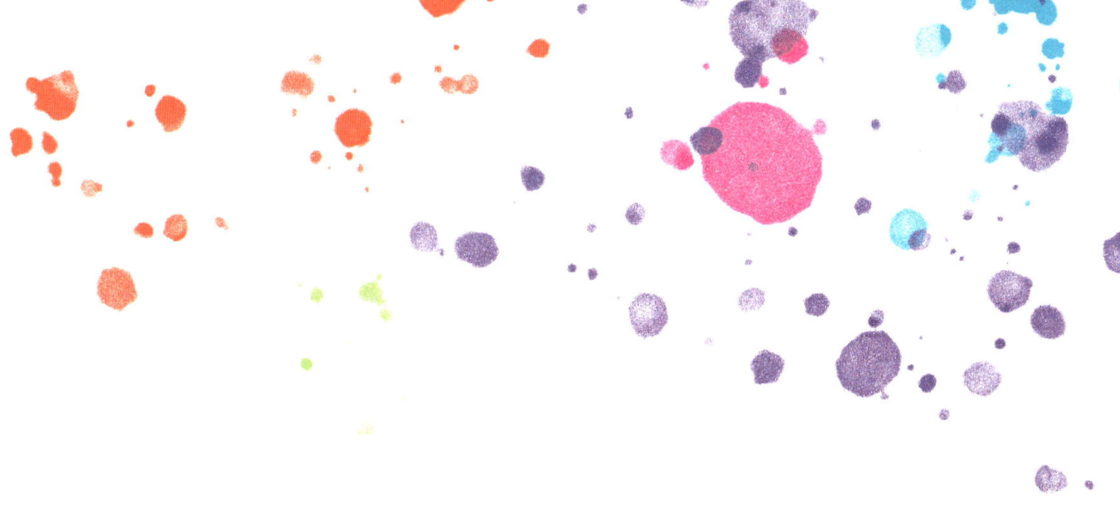

081

Three wishes

Try this when
you need to clarify
your priorities

You will need
Paper, markers, coloured pencils

15 minutes

Draw a magical genie lamp and write
three wishes you would love to come
true as soon as possible. Notice what you
have prioritized.

SELF-REFLECTION What priorities stand
out for you? Are they very different to the
current or past versions of yourself? If
they are, do you think you need to start
acting differently now in order to get
where you want to be?

Part of who you are is what you want to become

The gap between who you are
today and your future self can be
bridged with self-awareness and
intentionality. When you reflect
on who you want to become, you
become clear about your current
dreams, values, and priorities.
This information gives you
purpose, direction, and
motivation to do things in the
present moment that will affect
future outcomes, which is a
powerful tool for thriving and
for your personal wellbeing.

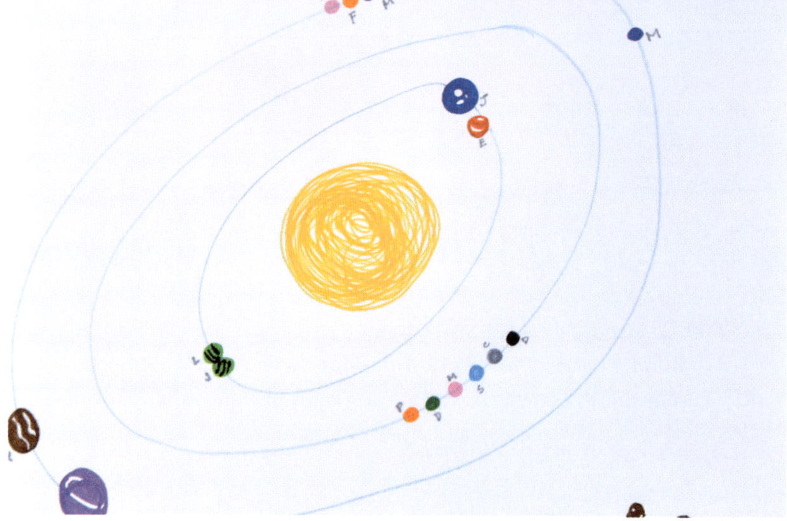

082

Family solar system

Try this when
you want to explore your
family dynamics

You will need
Paper, coloured pencils

20 minutes

Draw your family or social circle as celestial bodies,
such as planets, stars, and moons. Consider who
shines the brightest in your life, who orbits closest
to you, and who is furthest away when comparing
values and beliefs. Reflect on how distance, size, and
placement can depict the influence they exert over
your personality.

SELF-REFLECTION How did this exercise feel for you?
Did you note a strong presence of certain members?
What does that mean for your personality?

083

The dinner table

Try this when
you want to reflect who
matters most to you

You will need
Paper, coloured pencils

20 minutes

Draw your family's (both blood and chosen) dinner
table from your perspective – either as you were
growing up or as it is now. You can draw people or
use symbols to represent them.

SELF-REFLECTION Who is at the table? Who isn't? What
are people doing? What influence do they have on
the way you are and your personal wellbeing? Have
these people always accepted you as you are?

084

Your culture

Try this when
you want to explore
what shapes your identity

You will need
Paper, markers, coloured
pencils, mixed media

20 minutes

We can belong to various diverse cultures (relating to race, sex, gender, age, disability, and socioeconomic class, for example) and many of our beliefs and the way we experience feelings are shaped by them. What cultures do you belong to? Identify a colour for each of the groups mentioned above, then create an abstract piece that reflects how these colours interact. Do they blend smoothly, overlap, or stay separate?

SELF-REFLECTION Looking at how much space each colour occupies, do you believe there are cultural influences that shape your concept of yourself? Which parts are you most proud of and why?

085

Your heritage
self-portrait

Try this when
you want to connect with
your cultural identity

You will need
Paper, coloured pencils,
watercolours, paintbrushes

30 minutes

Create a self-portrait that represents your cultural identity – including not just your physical appearance, but also symbols, colours, and imagery that reflect your heritage, traditions, values, or experiences. You can incorporate elements from your upbringing, favourite foods, music, or traditions.

SELF-REFLECTION What elements did you include, and why are they meaningful to you? How has your cultural identity influenced the way you see yourself? Are there aspects of your heritage you feel deeply connected to or disconnected from?

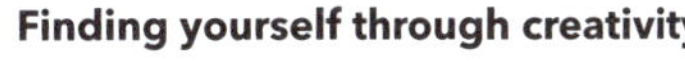

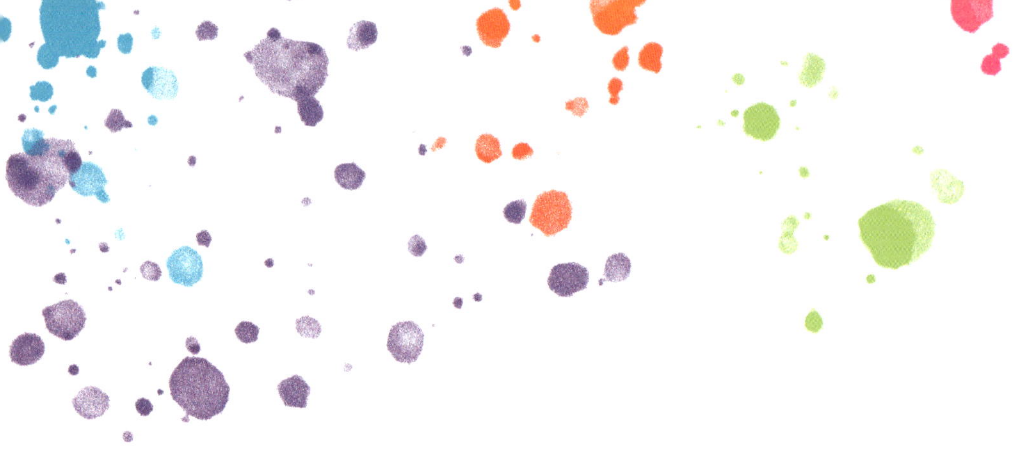

086

My personal quilt

Try this when
you want to connect with your roots

You will need
Paper, markers, coloured pencils,
watercolours, paintbrushes

30 minutes

Draw the outline of a quilt. It can be a
simple rectangle with squares inside,
including as many rows as you like. Fill
each section with meaningful symbols,
colours, and patterns to represent
different aspects of your cultural
influences - such as family, language,
traditions, personal experiences, or
particular places that have shaped you.

SELF-REFLECTION Do you feel protected
by and proud of your heritage? What
cultural threads feel the strongest in your
life? Are there influences that feel missing
or disconnected? Why?

087

My heritage map

Try this when
you want to celebrate your heritage

You will need
Paper, markers, coloured pencils,
watercolours, paintbrushes

30 minutes

Draw a map that represents your cultural
heritage - where your family comes from,
what influences have shaped your
ancestral history, and where you feel you
are now. Include meaningful places,
historical events, people, experiences, or
transitions that have been significant in
your family's cultural development.

SELF-REFLECTION What key experiences
have shaped your family history? How
have your cultural perspectives evolved
over time? Where do you feel most at
home, culturally speaking?

088

Favourite dish

Try this when
you want to discover
new influences

You will need
Paper, pencil, watercolours,
paintbrushes

20 minutes

Draw a plate containing a meal that you love. Where did this dish originate? How does it make you feel? Describe in writing what this dish can tell you about your own cultural background, identity, or influences.

SELF-REFLECTION Did the dish you chose stem from your own culture? If it didn't, how did you connect with this particular dish? What does this meal represent to you beyond physical nourishment?

089

Cultural soundtrack

Try this when
you want to explore your
personal story

You will need
Device for playing music,
paper, pencil, markers

30 minutes

Play three of your favourite songs and create art in response to what you are listening to. Try to think about how the music connects you to your different cultural identities. Use colours, symbols, or abstract shapes to express the emotions and memories tied to the music.

SELF-REFLECTION What songs or genres feel like home to you? Why? How has music influenced your understanding of your culture or identity? Are there any musical traditions you've embraced, rejected, or rediscovered over time?

090

Personal symbol

Try this when
you need a reminder of
your power

You will need
Paper, coloured pencils

15 minutes

Use this art experience to empower yourself. Draw an outline of your hand by tracing around it on a piece of paper. Inside the hand, create a design containing meaningful shapes, symbols, and colours to represent your most powerful self.

SELF-REFLECTION What elements did you include, and what do they represent? How do these symbols capture your personality or values? How did adding a symbolic design to your hand make you feel? Did it empower you?

Turning emotions into art

Emotions are often complex and can be difficult to put into words. However, art helps us express them authentically through colour, shape, and movement without needing to explain or justify them. In this chapter we explore how to manage our emotions by becoming self-aware and learning to identify, accept, and positively express them.

091

Emotional colour palette

Try this when
you want to express your feelings

You will need
Paper, coloured markers

10 minutes

Fold a sheet of paper horizontally, then vertically, to create four squares. Choose a colour that represents happiness and fill in the first square to show how you think happiness would move, such as twirls and jumps. Now pick a second colour to represent anger and reflect how it might move in the second square – perhaps jagged spikes. For your third square, select a colour for sadness. Maybe this moves slowly and barely touches the surface. Finally, choose a colour that represents peace and make soothing movements, such as gentle ripples, in the last square. The movement could follow the rhythm of your breath.

SELF-REFLECTION Were you able to find the rhythms of your own feelings? Were some feelings harder to draw than others? Could this be a sign that some emotions are more difficult for you to feel than others?

Express emotions through movement

The previous exercise helps you express emotions through colour and movement. Emotions live in the body, and while we often describe them with words, they naturally emerge through small physical gestures, like clenching a fist in anger or raising your eyebrows with surprise. Using movement to express emotions allows you to connect with them more authentically, making it easier to experience and release them in a healthy way.

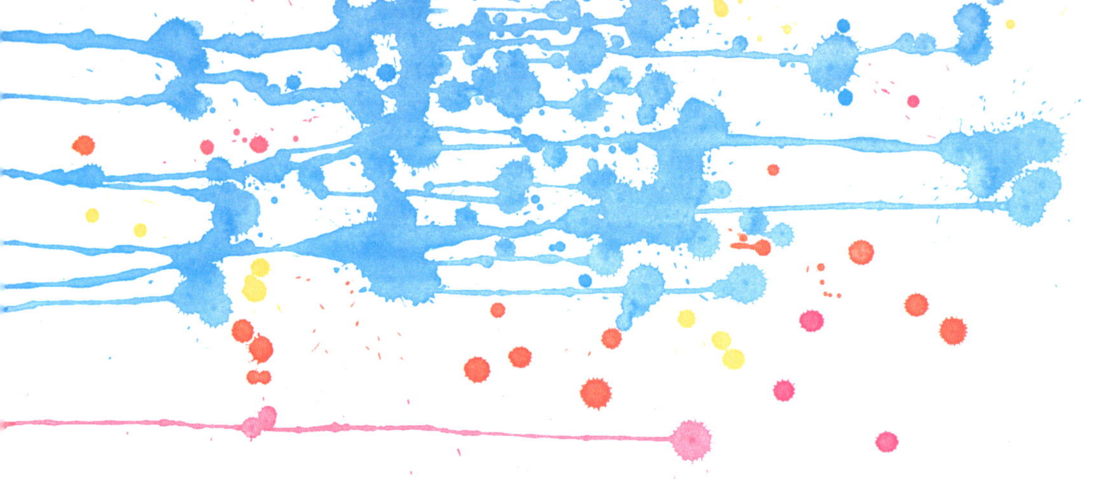

092

Emotional gradient (comfortable feelings)

Try this when
you want to explore the intensity
of your positive emotions

You will need
Paper, coloured pencils

20 minutes

Draw three columns and give each
column one of the following headings:
Happiness, Calm, Love. Then create
a colour gradient that represents the
intensity of each, from light to dark.
For example, with happiness you might
be content (light) or thrilled (darker).

SELF-REFLECTION Can you notice the
intensity of your feelings when you are
experiencing them? Are there things
you do that can take you from one end
of the spectrum to the other?

093

Emotional gradient (uncomfortable feelings)

Try this when
you want to explore the intensity
of your difficult emotions

You will need
Paper, coloured pencils

20 minutes

Again, draw three columns and give each
column one of the following headings:
Anger, Sadness, Fear. Then create a
colour gradient that represents the
intensity of each, from light to dark. For
example, with anger, you can be merely
irritated (lightest) or furious (very dark).

SELF-REFLECTION Is the intensity different
when you experience uncomfortable
emotions than with comfortable feelings?
Are there specific ones you experience
more often than others?

094

Emotional body map 1.0

Try this when
you want to explore how emotions impact your body

You will need
Paper, coloured pencils

20 minutes

Unexpressed emotions can turn into physical symptoms such as headaches, stomach problems, or muscle tension. Draw or print out an outline of a body and use different colours or lines to mark where you physically feel emotion in your body.

SELF-REFLECTION Were you able to identify where emotion is experienced in your body? Can you recognize whether some of these areas usually give you any physical health difficulties?

095

Symbolic meaning

Try this when
you want to reflect on your perception of emotions

You will need
Paper, pencil, coloured pencils

10 minutes

Even though emotions reside in the body, they also take shape in our thoughts and perceptions. First draw a symbol to represent each of these feelings: happiness, sadness, anger, fear, and calm. When you are finished, colour them in.

SELF-REFLECTION Did you notice any patterns of colour in your drawings? Can you start to identify the personal colour palette choices you associate with different emotions? How do the symbols you chose reflect the way you perceive each emotion?

096

Emotional body map 2.0

Try this when
you want to explore where emotions live in your body

You will need
Paper, coloured pencils

20 minutes

Draw or print out an outline of a body, then use the different symbols you created in the above exercise to identify where you physically feel each of those emotions in your body. For example, you might experience fear in the pit of your stomach, or sadness as a heaviness in your chest.

SELF-REFLECTION Were you able to identify where particular emotions live in your body? Can you use this knowledge as a way to understand what you might be feeling moving forward?

097

Feel better plan

Try this when
you need to remember what
lifts your spirits

You will need
Paper, coloured pencils, markers

15 minutes

Draw an outline of your hand by tracing around it. Inside the hand, write or draw things that help you feel better. It might be exercising, chatting with family and friends, or being outside in nature. Keep this drawing somewhere visible to remind you that there are many things you can do to help yourself when you are feeling low.

SELF-REFLECTION How often do you do these activities? Have you neglected them lately? Make sure you are engaging in pursuits that help boost your mood as a self-care practice.

098

Feeling through texture

Try this when
you feel tender about your emotions

You will need
Cardboard, glue, scissors, paint, paintbrushes, toilet paper, salt

30 minutes

On a piece of cardboard, use different brush strokes, pressure, and layered materials to represent textures that match your emotional state, such as rough for frustrated or smooth for peaceful. If you are comfortable with messy art, try mixing glue and water with toilet paper for added texture, or sprinkling salt on top of paint for a crystallized effect. If you aren't comfortable, then try scratching and poking holes in the surface of the cardboard using scissors for a tactile experience. Once dry or ready, paint over the whole thing to further explore your feelings through colour.

SELF-REFLECTION Was creating textures overwhelming for you, or did it feel grounding? Could engaging with your senses help you to emotionally regulate? Might a soft texture represent a yearning for comfort? Could a rough one express a need for clear boundaries or self-protection?

More healthy coping skills, please!

Try this when
you want to make positive coping skills part of your routine

You will need
Sticky notes, coloured pencils, markers

15 minutes

Choose five activities that you would like to add to your routine, then draw a symbol for each of these on separate sticky notes. For example, you might draw a notebook to indicate journalling, or a thought cloud to depict taking time for positive affirmations. Place them around your house to remind you to engage with them at least once a week.

SELF-REFLECTION Did you choose activities that are easy to integrate into your life? Or are they more challenging? Try scheduling time for them on your phone calendar as well.

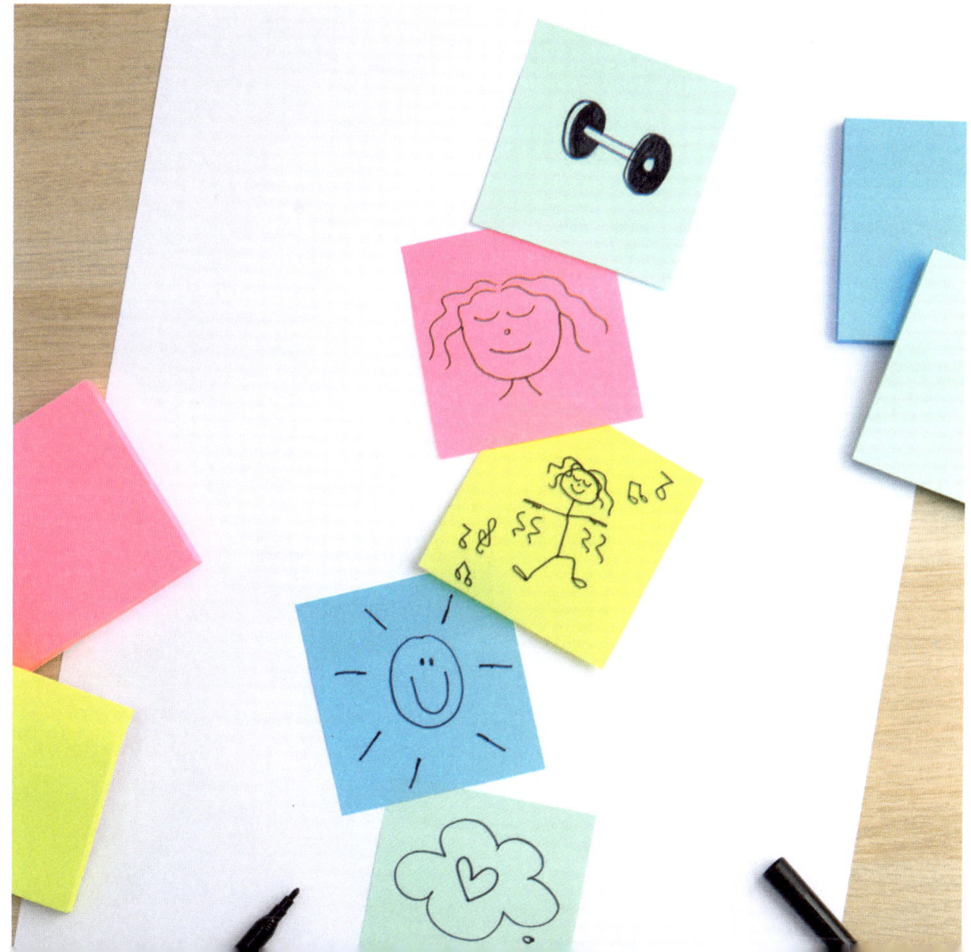

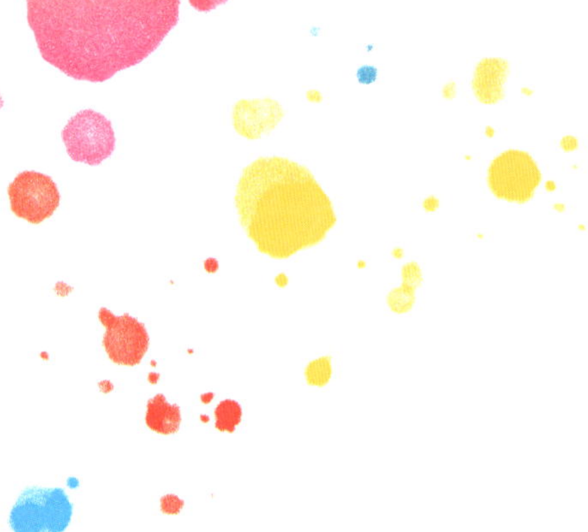

100

Free scribble part 1

Try this when
you want to express your
feelings freely

You will need
Paper, pencil or marker

3 minutes

Close your eyes, take a deep breath, and
scribble freely for 30 seconds on a sheet
of paper. Allow yourself to go as fast or
slow as you need to. When the time is
up, open your eyes.

SELF-REFLECTION Were you able to
create freely, or were you scared of the
outcome? If perfectionism is getting in
the way, remember the lessons learned in
the previous section. Were you going fast
or slow? Could this represent a rhythm
your body is craving to be in?

101

Free scribble part 2

Try this when
you feel unclear about your
emotional state

You will need
Paper, pencil, coloured pencils

10 minutes

Take the scribble you made in the
previous exercise and transform it into
a meaningful image or pattern. Look for
any symbols that emerge naturally (like
when you're spotting shapes in clouds)
or highlight specific areas, such as
intersections of the lines, by adding
colour or definition.

SELF-REFLECTION Did you find particular
symbols that might be representing your
current emotional state? Look at the
colour choices you made: could the
palette be communicating any of the
feelings you are experiencing?

Self-soothing scribble

Try this when
you are in need of comfort

You will need
Music device, paper, watercolours, paintbrushes

5 minutes

This exercise can be useful for focusing on your body in order to distract yourself from a racing brain. Find a song or piece of music that you find soothing, then choose a colour that feels comforting to you. While the music is playing, allow your brush to draw the rhythm you are listening to in one continuous line. Let your hand be the guide to quieten your mind.

SELF-REFLECTION Were you able to focus on the sensory experience of listening and coordinating your body's movement? Or was your busy mind distracting you? This is an active meditation exercise, and these sometimes require practice, so don't give up – simply try again when you're ready.

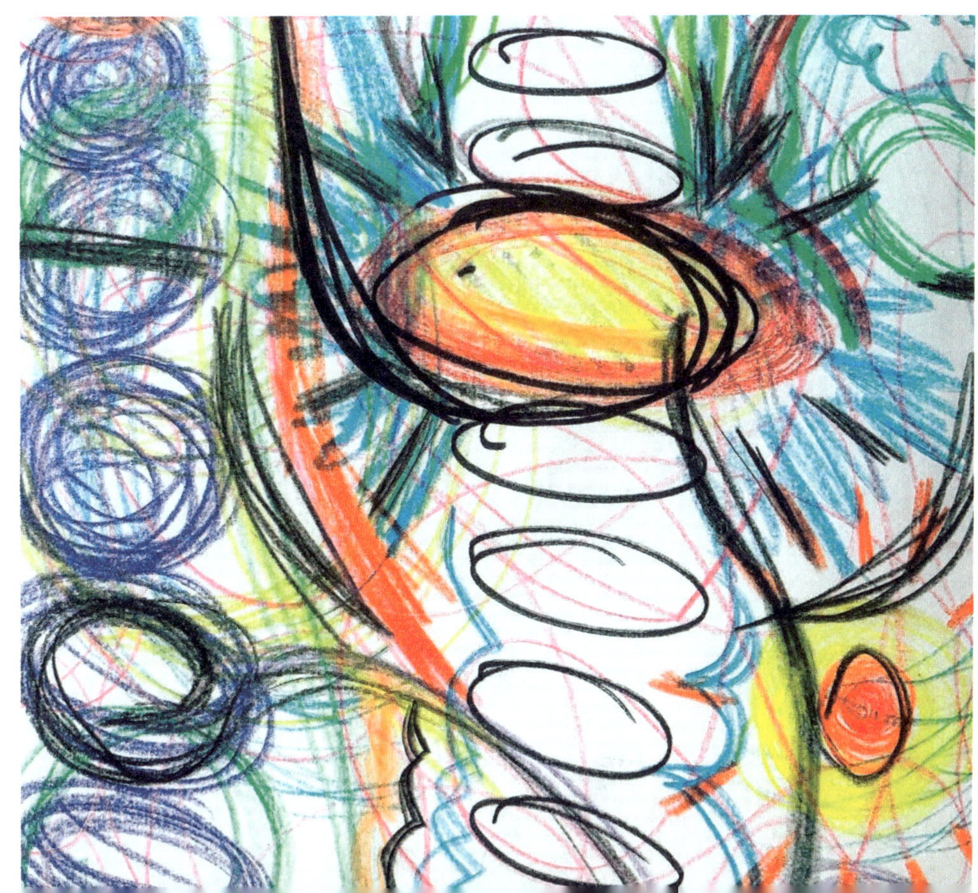

103

Breathing colours

Try this when
you want to quiet
your mind

You will need
Paper, two colours of
marker

5 minutes

This active meditation exercise can help with grounding. Take a different coloured marker in each hand, then draw circles or scribbles with one hand as you breathe in. When you breathe out, do the same but with the opposite hand. Keep going until your heart feels content.

SELF-REFLECTION Did using alternate hands help you to disconnect from your thoughts and focus on your breathing? Could this mean engaging in mindful movement can help calm your mind and reduce emotional discomfort? Would you consider trying activities like knitting or crocheting as an emotional coping tool?

104

Soothing patterns

Try this when
you need to regulate
your emotions

You will need
Sticky note, pen, coloured
pencils

5 minutes

Fill a sticky note or a paper similar in size with repetitive marks, doodles, or patterns using a pen or pencils in comforting colours. This intentionally slow rhythmic movement can help regulate your emotions.

SELF-REFLECTION How did it feel to slow down? Did it come naturally, or did it feel forced? Could this be a sign you need to slow down in your own life as well?

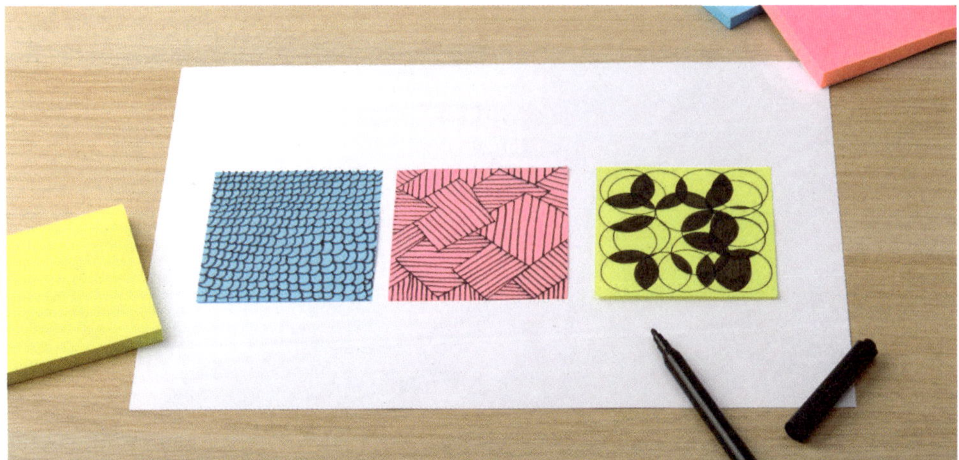

105

Forbidden feelings

Try this when
you feel emotionally
invalidated

You will need
Paper, coloured pencils

20 minutes

Draw an open book. On the left-hand page, write or illustrate the "unspoken rules" your family has about emotions. For example, "We don't show anger" or "Always be cheerful". On the right-hand page, rewrite these rules in a way that allows for more emotional freedom, such as "Anger is a valid feeling", or "Crying shows strength". Decorate this page, adding new thoughts around emotional liberation, using colours and symbols to express these healthier guidelines.

SELF-REFLECTION What emotions have you struggled to express? How has that shaped how you handle your emotions today? What would it feel like to fully embrace your emotions as valuable and necessary? How can you start doing that in small ways?

106

Feeling triggers

Try this when
you want to explore your
emotional triggers

You will need
Paper, coloured pencils

15 minutes

It is important to not only know what helps you feel better, but also to identify what triggers you. Draw the outline of three cages. Inside each cage, draw a different monster, then identify what trigger each monster represents. Is it a person, situation, or memory? Knowing what gets you emotionally shaken is important so that next time it shows up, you are in control of it, and not the other way around.

SELF-REFLECTION Were the monsters scary? Or did they not look so bad once they were externalized and in a cage? Will you be able to stop them next time they try to get to you?

REMEMBER If this exercise feels overwhelming, try the previous self-soothing exercises to help you regulate. Remember, if you are feeling disturbed, you can always reach out to an expert for further exploration of the issue.

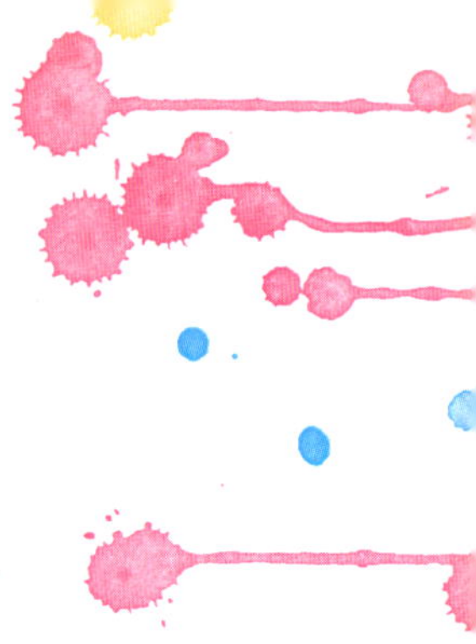

107
Feeling through symbols

Try this when
your emotions are holding you back

You will need
Paper, pencil, coloured pencils

10 minutes

Think of an emotion you are currently experiencing. Now look online or in a book or magazine for an image that represents it. Try copying that image onto a piece of paper. It doesn't have to look exactly the same, the aim here is self-expression.

SELF-REFLECTION Did you experience an emotional release once you saw your final image? Seeing our emotions externalized can be very liberating. Or were you so focused on the quality of the drawing that you were left feeling the same? Could you be struggling with some self-limiting perfectionism?

108
Emotional colouring page part 1

Try this when
you want to make space for all of your emotions

You will need
Predesigned image to colour in, coloured pencils, markers

15 minutes

Make space for feelings to be present. Identify at least three different emotions from pp.12–13 that demonstrate how you are feeling today. Assign a colour to each emotion, then use these to colour in with.

SELF-REFLECTION Was your hand tense or relaxed when colouring? Were you working slowly or quickly? What colours stand out the most? Could this mean that those feelings are more dominant? How could you make space for all of your feelings?

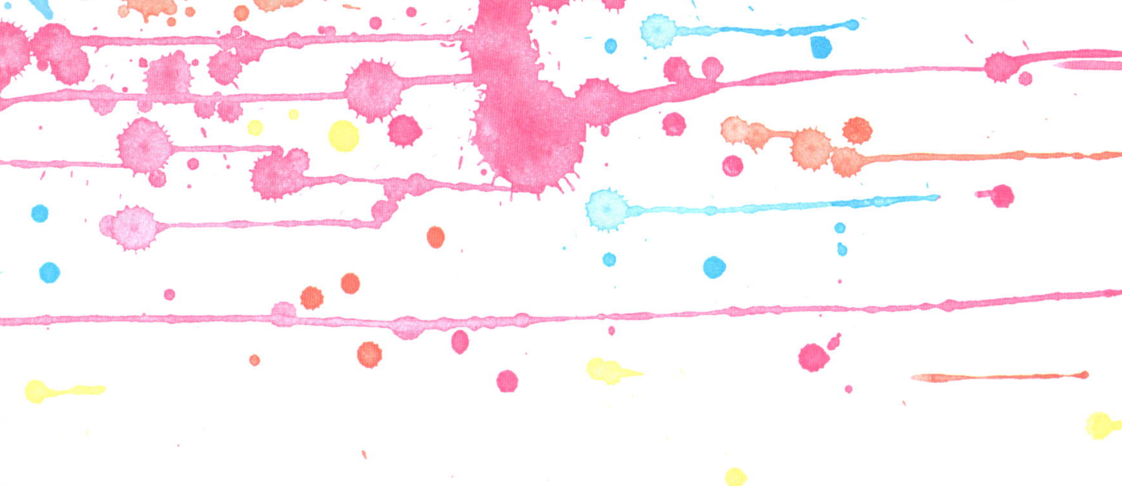

109

Emotional colouring page part 2

Try this when
you need to externalize your feelings

You will need
Predesigned image to colour in, coloured pencils, markers

15 minutes

If you have identified certain colour choices or palettes to represent specific feelings, try using those on a colouring page. You could, for example, only use cheerful yellow tones to colour in. Notice how using these colours makes you feel. Consider the pace of your colouring: is it slow and smooth, or quick and intense?

SELF-REFLECTION Were you able to be intentional with the colour choice and movement to help you express an emotion? How did the colours and pace influence your emotional state?

110

Inside-out silhouette

Try this when
you want to stop hiding how you feel

You will need
Paper, pencil, markers, coloured pencils

20 minutes

Trace the outline of your hand on a piece of paper. Inside the hand, draw or write what you are feeling internally. Around the outside of the hand, depict how you show up to the world. For example, you might write "sad" or "lonely" inside the hand, but "bubbly" outside.

SELF-REFLECTION Compare both sides. If they are very different, could you be masking your emotions? Bottling up your feelings can lead to a worsening mental health condition. Could you consider talking to a specialist?

How art can make us feel

Mood is a persistent emotional state that influences how we perceive and respond to the world. Unlike fleeting emotions, moods are subtle and pervasive, shaping our general outlook over hours or even days without always having a clear cause. Think about it for a second. If you are in a "good" mood, you will be more tolerant of things happening around you. However, if you are in a "bad" one, you may be less patient. Moods can exert a big influence on the way we feel on a daily basis, and this is called "affect".

Try this when
you want to understand your
emotional state

30 minutes

What are mood and affect?

The difference between mood and affect lies in their duration and expression. Affect is more about the immediate, observable expression of emotions in the moment, while mood is more sustained and internal, influencing emotions over time without always being outwardly noticeable.

111 Mood colour flow

You will need
Paper, watercolours, paintbrushes

Choose three colours that represent your mood over the past week. Use a brush to wet a blank piece of paper, then fill the damp page with your three colours. Watch them spread and notice how they interact with one another. Let the sheet dry and save it for the next exercise.

112 Moods and affect

You will need
Previously created mood colour flow art, coloured pencils

Using your previous mood art as the base, consider how you are feeling right now. Think of the kind of day you are having and what emotions are present within you (see pp.12–13 for inspiration). Once you have identified your feelings, either draw an abstract representation of your emotions using colour and movement, or use symbols to represent your current affect. Choose whatever calls to you in the moment.

SELF-REFLECTION What patterns did you notice in your art? Are there colours or images that repeat themselves? How does it feel to look at your current affect on your mood art? Are they similar, or is there a mismatch? For example, is your mood colour art indicating sadness, but your affect shows you are feeling lonely? Use this to identify how you are doing, and if you see anything that concerns you, maybe suggestive of overwhelm, consider asking for help.

113

Lines and trends

Try this when
you want to check in
on your mood

You will need
Paper, coloured pencils,
collage images, mixed media

30 minutes

Draw a line across the length of the paper to use as a timeline. Divide it into days of the week, then start adding colour, images, and words to represent how you felt each day.

SELF-REFLECTION What patterns do you notice in your art? Are there colour or images that repeat themselves? Use this to identify how you are doing. If there is anything that concerns you, such as worsening feelings of despair or rapid mood changes, consider seeking help from a specialist.

114

My weather report

Try this when
you want to explore your
emotional patterns

You will need
Paper, pencil, coloured
pencils, markers

30 minutes

Draw seven rectangles in a row, like a template for a weekly weather forecast, and label each with a day of the week. Instead of numbers or words, use meteorological symbols to represent your emotions for each day – sunny for joy, cloudy for uncertainty, rain for sadness, or a thunderstorm for anger.

SELF-REFLECTION Did you notice any patterns emerging? Were there specific reasons for the emotions you represented? If you had sunny days, were there things you did that you could repeat again soon?

115

30 heart check-ins

Try this when
you want to deepen your
emotional awareness

You will need
Paper, coloured pencils

5 minutes

Learn to check in with yourself through this easy practice. Draw 30 (or 31) hearts to represent days of the month. For each day, colour in a heart using a shade that reflects your emotional state. At the end of the month, look for patterns and possible connections between your emotions and daily experiences.

SELF-REFLECTION How did it feel to have daily check-ins with yourself? Was it hard or easy to give space for your feelings to exist? Was it useful to pay attention, even if only a little, to acknowledge where your heart was instead of just your thoughts?

116

Emotional container

Try this when
you want to express your
emotions in a healthy way

You will need
Empty box, paint,
paintbrushes, mixed media

20 minutes

Creating a container to hold all the negative feelings happening inside us, allows us to externalize them in a safe way. Paint the outside of an empty box with colours that represent strength and stability, adding any decorations that feel grounding. Once dry, fill the inside of the box with colours, shapes, or words that express overwhelming emotions. Store this box in a secure place, or keep its contents private by using symbols or colours instead of words, and use it as a safe space to release your feelings when needed.

SELF-REFLECTION How does it feel to have an external container for what is happening inside you? Did it bring any relief or new insights? How might using this box regularly help you process difficult emotions in a healthy way?

117

Bridging the gap

Try this when
you want to improve your
emotional state

You will need
Paper, markers, coloured
pencils

15 minutes

Sometimes, using imagination can help you achieve distance from uncomfortable feelings. On one side of a piece of paper, draw a symbol representing your current emotional state. On the other side, depict how you would like to feel. Draw a road between them, then on the road, use colours, symbols, or words to represent what you could do to get from one end to the other.

SELF-REFLECTION Was it easy to find things to do that can help you get from one emotional state to the other? Or was it difficult? If you are having a hard time improving your emotional state, consider speaking to an art therapist or other professional.

118

Adult tantrum

Try this when
you need to release
bottled-up emotions

You will need
Paper, markers

15 minutes

Draw a large speech bubble, and inside it draw
or write anything that is bothering you. Remember,
this is for your eyes only. When you are done, tear
the paper into very small pieces and throw it away
– nobody needs to know about it.

SELF-REFLECTION Were you able to let yourself go and
express all of your thoughts? Or did you hold back?
Did you feel a physical release?

119

Tangled feelings

Try this when
you feel confused about
your emotional state

You will need
Paper, coloured pencils

20 minutes

Sometimes, mixed feelings can be harder to identify
if we are overthinking them. When you don't know
how you feel, draw an empty jar, then select five
different colours and scribble inside the jar, layering
all of the colours on top of each other. Now draw five
straight lines on a separate piece of paper, each in
a different colour, and try to identify what emotion
each colour could be representing for you right now
(see pp.12–13 for inspiration).

SELF-REFLECTION Did the colours help bring clarity
over your emotional state? What surprised you most
about the emotions you connected with each colour?

120

Affirmation art

Try this when
you need guidance to improve
your emotional wellbeing

You will need
Paper, watercolours,
paintbrushes

20 minutes

Having wisdom around you can help you to
deal with difficult emotions. Write a self-soothing
affirmation or inspiring quote in bold letters, then
surround it with colours, symbols, or imagery that
reinforces its message.

SELF-REFLECTION What kind of wisdom did you
depict? Is it a phrase that highlights your values and
personal strengths, or reminds you of better times?
How easy will it be to introduce this concept into
your daily life?

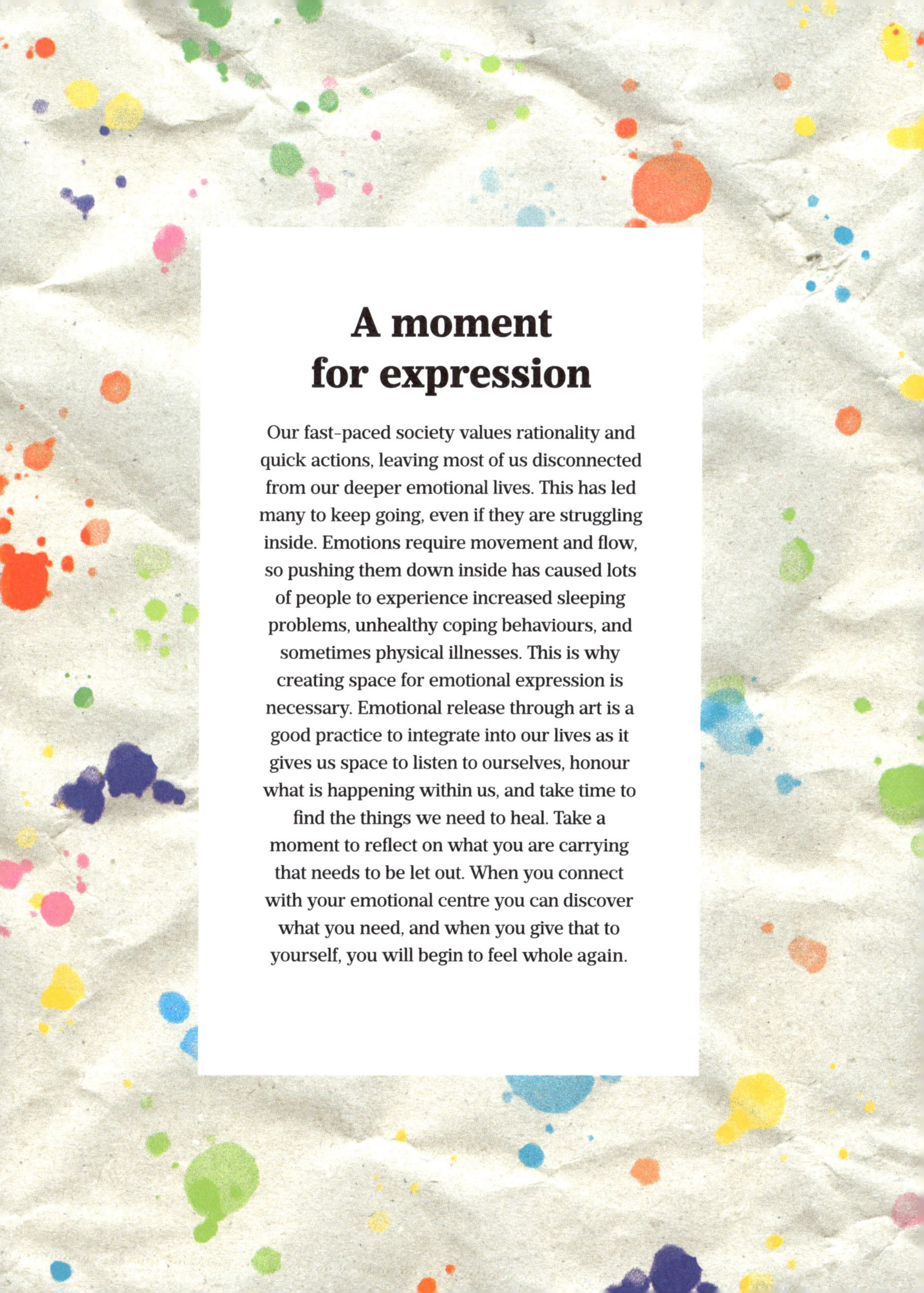

A moment for expression

Our fast-paced society values rationality and quick actions, leaving most of us disconnected from our deeper emotional lives. This has led many to keep going, even if they are struggling inside. Emotions require movement and flow, so pushing them down inside has caused lots of people to experience increased sleeping problems, unhealthy coping behaviours, and sometimes physical illnesses. This is why creating space for emotional expression is necessary. Emotional release through art is a good practice to integrate into our lives as it gives us space to listen to ourselves, honour what is happening within us, and take time to find the things we need to heal. Take a moment to reflect on what you are carrying that needs to be let out. When you connect with your emotional centre you can discover what you need, and when you give that to yourself, you will begin to feel whole again.

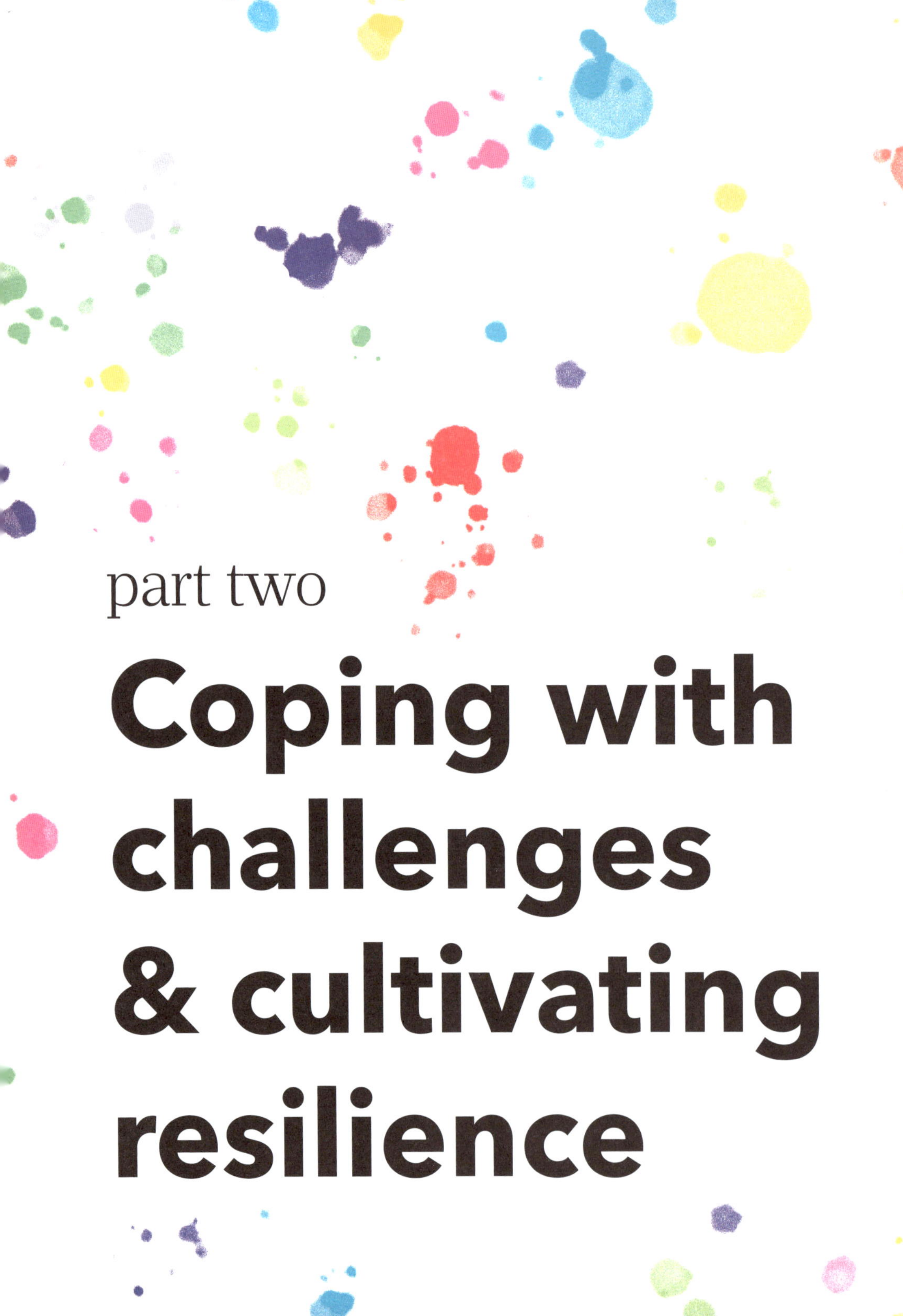

part two

Coping with challenges & cultivating resilience

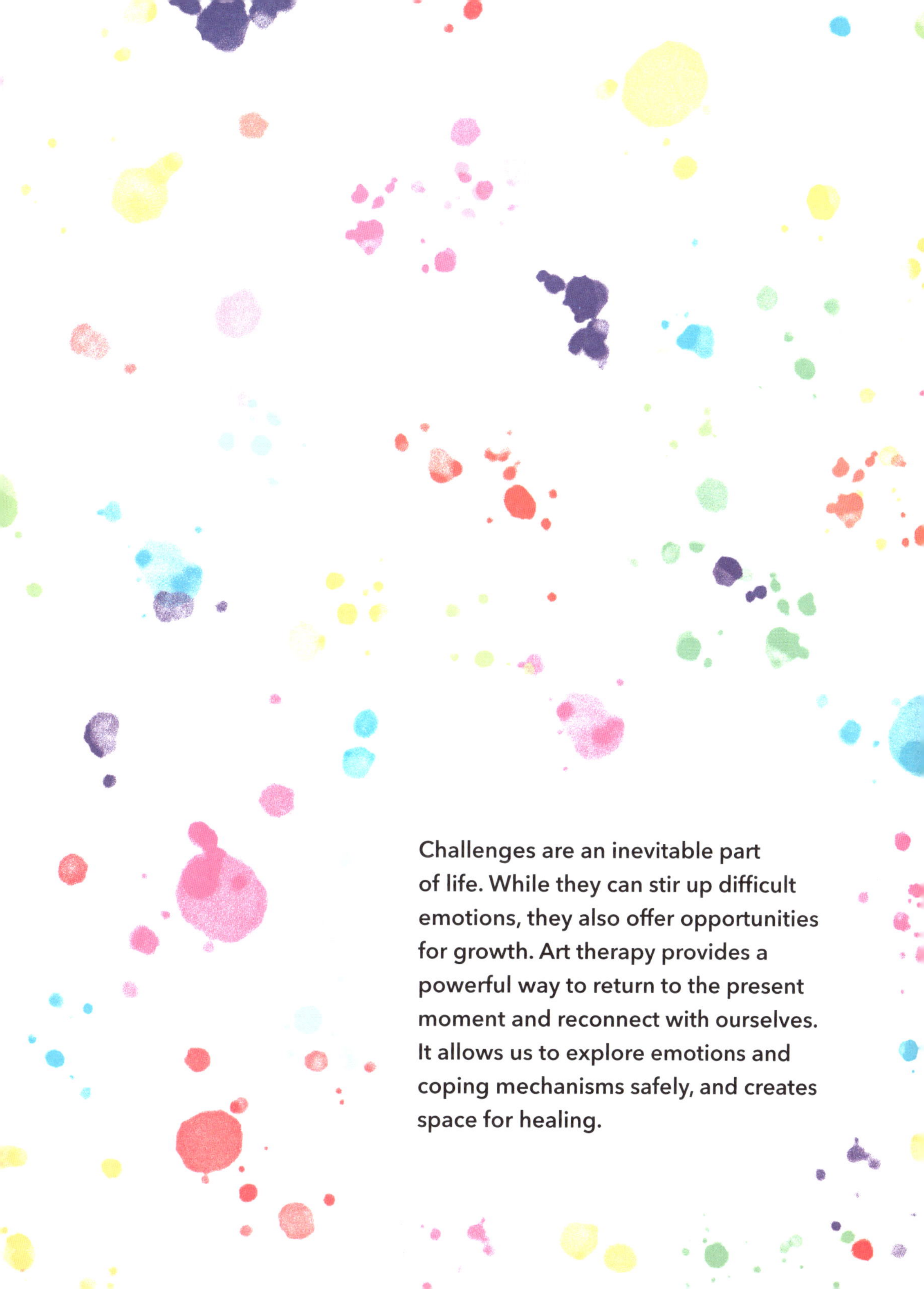

Challenges are an inevitable part of life. While they can stir up difficult emotions, they also offer opportunities for growth. Art therapy provides a powerful way to return to the present moment and reconnect with ourselves. It allows us to explore emotions and coping mechanisms safely, and creates space for healing.

Releasing fear & finding courage

Fear isn't inherently bad – it's a natural response to perceived threats, designed to drive us into action. When we take the time to understand and process fear, it can help us build resilience – the willingness to act and draw strength from our values and character, even in moments of vulnerability. Art therapy offers a safe and supportive space to do this.

121

Getting to know fear

Try this when
you want to explore the
depths of your fear

You will need
Paper, watercolours,
paintbrush

20 minutes

Choose a colour to represent your fear. Think of a time you felt a little afraid and paint the right-hand side of the page with a soft hue of your chosen colour. Then think of a time when you felt extremely scared and paint the left-hand side with the darkest hue. Starting from the dark side, fill in the middle section, creating a gradient with the paint getting lighter as you move across the page. While you are connecting both sides together, reflect on how fear, just like all feelings, has different levels of intensity.

SELF-REFLECTION If you are experiencing fear right now, can you tell where you are on the scale? Are you in the darkest section or in a lighter colour? Does any section feel more manageable or familiar? If you could add a colour to symbolize courage, what would it be and where would you place it?

122

The story of fear

Try this when
fear feels overwhelming

You will need
Paper, pencil, coloured
pencils

20 minutes

Fear can be an overwhelming sensation, so it's important to find ways to keep it under control. Fold a piece of paper lengthwise into three sections. In the middle section, draw a fear you are currently experiencing, allowing it to exist. In the left-hand section, draw what caused this fear to appear. In the section on the right, draw a strategy to help control the fear.

SELF-REFLECTION How does your story shift when you take control of the narrative? How does re-imagining your fear help you approach it differently in real life? What needs to happen for your strategy to become a reality?

123

The friendly monster

Try this when
you want to shift your
perspective on fear

You will need
Paper, pencil, coloured
pencils, markers

20 minutes

Rather than seeing your fear as menacing, view it as a protector. Imagine your fear as a character or creature and draw it. Instead of making it a scary monster, try adding features to make it friendlier, such as a smile or soft eyes. Name your character and take a moment to think about how it may help you see fear as favourable and protective rather than something to be afraid of.

SELF-REFLECTION How does it feel to envision your fear as a character? If this character had a message for you, what would it say? What would happen if you added another feature, such as a superhero cape or a mask, to make it even less intimidating and more protective?

124

Introducing Mr Monster

Try this when
you want to make fear feel
more manageable

You will need
Paper, pencil, coloured
pencils, markers

30 minutes

Storytelling can make exploring your emotions less intimidating. Using your fear character from the previous exercise, design a comic book page introducing them to the world. Answer these questions: what's their name? What do they like and dislike? What makes them strong? What makes them weak? As you develop the story, think about the moments when your fear feels strongest. Is it just before a presentation, or when test results are due? Also reflect on what weakens it. Perhaps you've noticed that taking deep breaths, exercising, or talking to a loved one alleviates your fear for a while.

SELF-REFLECTION When is your fear character the strongest? Did you notice any patterns? Are these moments real threats or perceived ones? How do you feel giving your fear a personality change, and how do you relate to it? Does it seem more manageable or less intimidating?

125
What hides in the shadows

Try this when
you want to explore where your
fears come from

You will need
Paper, pencil, timer

15 minutes

Draw a human figure nearly the size of
the sheet of paper, then draw the shadow
it casts. The shadow symbolizes the fears
that you carry. What are you afraid of?
Where could these fears have come
from? Set a timer for 3 minutes and,
using the free-writing technique (p.90),
write down in the shadow area all the
thoughts that come to mind. This is not
about confronting your fears, it's about
bringing them to awareness. Save this
drawing for the next exercise.

SELF-REFLECTION How hard was it to write
about your fears for 3 minutes without
stopping? Did any of these resonate
with you? Could this represent how
comfortable you are with sitting with
your fears? How do these fears show
up in your everyday life?

126
What lives in the light

Try this when
you are ready to stand up to
your fears

You will need
Drawing from previous exercise,
coloured pencils, marker

20 minutes

Take your drawing from the previous
exercise and read the fears that you
wrote in the shadow. Then using different
coloured pencils, write down strategies
inside the body that you could use to
face your fears. You can be as creative
as you like, such as defeating them in
an imaginary sword fight, or they can
be real-life coping skills, like taking
deep breaths before facing the fear, or
visualizing a happy place. Use a marker
to highlight strategies that feel most
empowering to you.

SELF-REFLECTION Was it easy to identify
coping strategies for your fears? Could
you use some of these in your own life
now? Are you already using any of
these strategies?

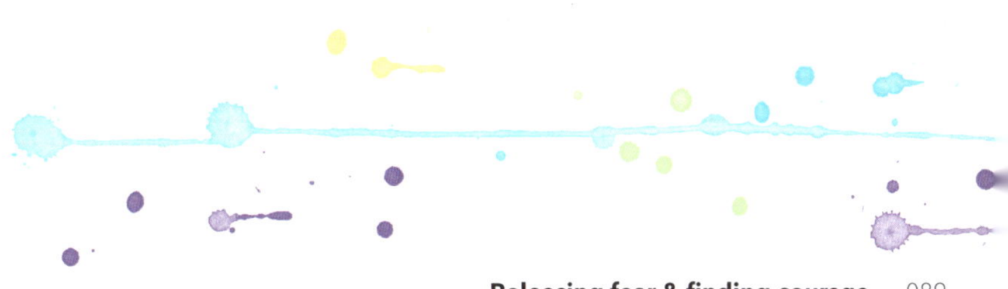

127
What are you afraid of?

Try this when
you want to get to the
heart of what scares you

You will need
Paper, pen, timer

20 minutes

Begin by drawing a slightly open door,
then turn the paper over and, using the
free-writing technique, write about your
fears for 10 minutes without stopping.

SELF-REFLECTION How open or closed
was your door? Could this represent how
open you are to seeing your fears? Did
your writing help you understand what
you may be afraid of?

Free-writing

Free-writing is a technique
where you note down whatever
comes to mind without
censoring or editing it, even if it
doesn't make sense for an alloted
amount of time. Writing without
hesitation can allow unconscious
thoughts and feelings to emerge.

128
The fear map part 1

Try this when
you want to explore
what you are afraid of

You will need
Paper, pencil, coloured
pencils, markers

30 minutes

Draw a map of your "fear world". This
could be an island, a maze, a mountain,
or a city. Then assign symbols to your
different fears. For example, a gloomy
forest could symbolize being frightened
of the dark, a desert may be a fear of
being alone, and a turbulent sea might
represent self-doubt. Try connecting the
different parts of your fear landscape
with roads, rivers, or trails to show how
they could be linked to one another.

SELF-REFLECTION What do you notice
about your fears? Are some smaller
or bigger than others? Did you notice
any changes in how you can relate to
your fears after seeing them in front
of you? Could some of your fears be
interconnected, making them worse?

129

The fear map part 2

Try this when
you want to connect
with what feels safe

You will need
Paper, pencil, coloured
pencils, markers

20 minutes

When you explore your fear landscape, it's important to identify safe spaces. Try to represent your inner strengths or support systems by drawing them on your fear map. Maybe your meditation practice can look like a lighthouse, or a specific friend can be a bridge leading to a secure spot?

SELF-REFLECTION Are the places, people, or practices that help you feel better connected in the drawing? Or are they separated and isolated? Imagine you can draw a new path leading away from your fears. Where would it take you? How does it feel to look at your safe spaces? Did your fears become less threatening?

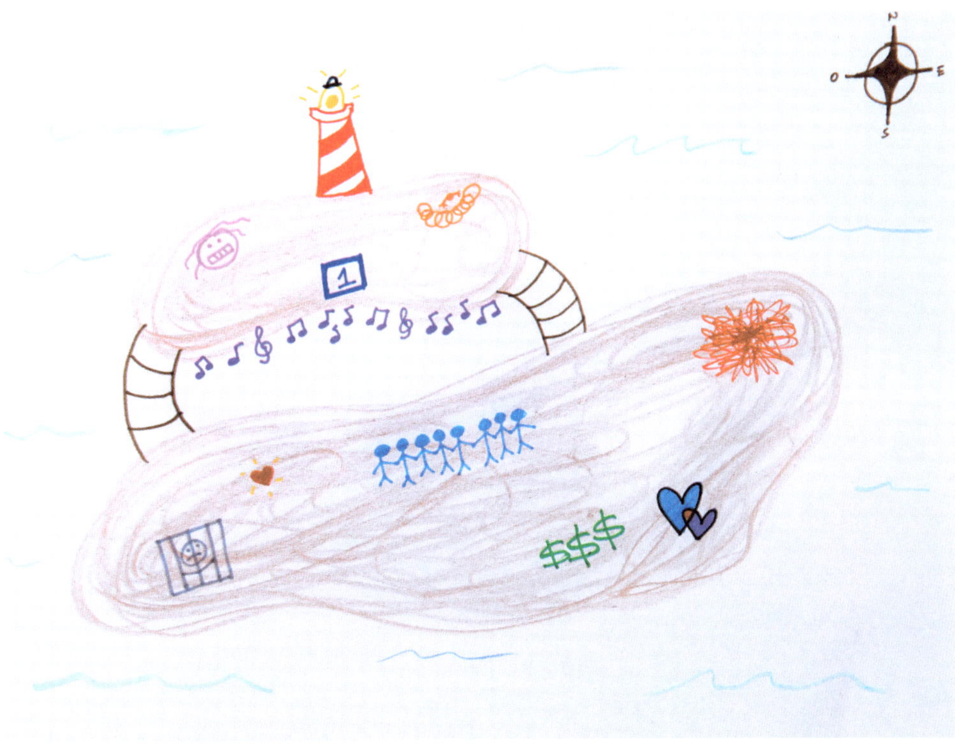

130

Fear in the body

Try this when
you want to practise sitting
with uncomfortable feelings

You will need
Paper, pencil, materials that
you find uncomfortable

30 minutes

Find a quiet space and check in with
your body. Notice where you feel fear
the most – it might be in your stomach,
lower back, or shoulders. If possible,
identify the physical sensations related
to fear, such as tension, tingling feelings,
or tightness. Then, visualize a symbol
emerging from the area you focused
on and draw it using materials you
identified on p.20 as provoking
discomfort. If you start to feel tense,
pause for a moment. If it's comfortable
to do so, close your eyes and breathe
slowly and deeply. Remind yourself that
you are safe and in control. If this feels
overwhelming, consider working with an
art therapist.

SELF-REFLECTION How does it feel to sit
with discomfort in a creative manner?
Was it a cathartic experience? Did you
notice a difference after taking some
slow, deep breaths?

131

Fear splotches

Try this when
you want to express your
feelings freely

You will need
Paper, paint, paintbrushes,
timer

20 minutes

Learning to express emotions in a
positive way is crucial for your mental
health. Choose a colour to represent
your fear, and use your brush at different
speeds to create splotches across the
whole page. Notice which pace feels
more aligned with your experience of
fear and how much pressure you use on
the brush. Is it light or strong? Is it slow
or fast? Evaluate which one reflects your
emotion better. Once you've found the
rhythm and pressure that you feel is right,
continue making splotches around the
page for 3 minutes. When you have
finished, take a deep breath to ground
yourself and release the emotion.

SELF-REFLECTION Were your brushstrokes
light and quick or strong and slow?
How did the speed and pressure of
your brushstrokes communicate your
experience of fear? Could this be a
reflection of your daily life? How did your
body feel before, during, and after the
activity? Did you notice any difference?

132

Scary story time part 1

Try this when
you are ready to
welcome your fears

You will need
Paper, pen, markers,
coloured pencils

30 minutes

Using the free-writing technique (p.90), write a story about something you are scared of, filling three pieces of paper. Allow yourself to write freely, even if phrases don't seem to be making sense. Continue writing without stopping. Once you have finished, draw an image that represents your story.

SELF-REFLECTION What emotions arise when you view your fears as something separate from yourself? Are they more or less intimidating? Does your drawing reveal the content of your story? Could this mean you are ready to share your fears with others, or do you want to keep this to yourself?

133

Scary story time part 2

Try this when
you are ready to take
control of your fears

You will need
Paper, pen, coloured pencils

30 minutes

Rewrite the story you just wrote and make all the changes you need to regain control of the narrative and your feelings about your fear. You might add new characters, construct a different ending, or have another beginning to the story. Once done, draw another image to represent your new story.

SELF-REFLECTION How did it feel to rewrite your own story? Did it change dramatically? Could this mean you are ready to transform your life story on your own, or do you need support? Remember, you can always change the things you don't like in your life.

Catharsis

If you find yourself in tears after any of the activities, don't worry, it's normal. This can occur when you sit with discomfort, as it can make your emotions more intense. Crying is your body's natural way of processing and releasing what you are feeling.

Navigating rough waters

Challenges are an inevitable part of life. They will appear unexpectedly and sometimes shake you to your core. However, through art, you can find ways to anchor yourself back to your centre and remind yourself that you are able to navigate any storm that strikes.

134 **Steering through storms**

You will need

Paper, art materials of your choice

Fear can arise when you are faced with difficult situations. Paint a boat sailing through a storm. Make sure to add sails, anchors, a motor, or any accessory that you think can help the boat steer through it. Save this art for the next exercise.

135 **All hands on deck**

You will need

Paper, art materials of your choice

Place the painting of the boat in front of you. On another piece of paper, draw the boat again, but consider how you could improve its safety. Think about how the different parts of the boat could represent the things that give you courage in your life. Could a new anchor be an intention that keeps you steady or a loved one that helps you stay grounded? Could the sails be your motivations or the people that push you in the right direction?

136 **Anchors aweigh**

You will need

Paper, pencil, coloured pencils, markers

Sticking to your core values can help you feel most aligned with yourself, serving as a compass that guides your behaviour when you are faced with challenges. Draw an anchor that could help your boat remain steady during the storm. Inside the anchor, write or draw the values (pp.10–13) that you are most proud of holding.

SELF-REFLECTION What do you notice about the storm? Do you think the boat will be able to survive the tempest? What do you notice about the second boat you drew? Did it need many modifications? Could this boat endure not only the current storm, but also future ones? Was it easy or difficult to identify your core values? Do you use these values to prioritize decisions in your life? Do you follow them, or do you feel that sometimes outside pressure makes you put them to one side?

137
Courageous self-portrait

Try this when
you need a reminder of
your inner bravery

You will need
Paper, pencil, coloured pencils

30 minutes

When we consciously choose courage
over avoidance, fear loses its power to
control us. Draw a portrait of yourself at
a time when you felt courageous, and
around it write what was happening in
your life and why you felt brave.

SELF-REFLECTION How did it feel to
reconnect with yourself at a time when
you felt brave? Was it easy or difficult to
embrace yourself at your best? Was the
moment you felt this way a long time
ago? Maybe it's time to reconnect with
that part of yourself again.

138
Personal hero

Try this when
you feel overwhelmed by self-doubt

You will need
Paper, photo of yourself to cut
out, pencil, coloured pencils,
scissors, glue

30 minutes

When you are fearful, it's easy for
self-doubt to creep in, so it's important to
remind yourself of what you have to give.
Take a moment to reflect on personal
strengths, such as creativity, empathy,
and patience, then identify at least five
you possess. Attach a photo of your
face to the top of a piece of paper, then
draw yourself as a superhero by adding
a body and suit. Imagine what kind of
superpowers your strengths could
give you.

SELF-REFLECTION Are you proud of the
superhero you've created? Do you think
this character can come to the rescue
when you are afraid?

139

Defining courage

Try this when
courage feels out of reach

You will need
Paper, magazine or image
printouts, scissors, glue

20 minutes

Make a collage depicting what courage looks like
to you. You can include specific representations of
actions or people that you think are brave. Notice
how realistic your representation of courage looks.

SELF-REFLECTION How practical are your expectations
of courage? Can you start incorporating some of the
behaviours you glued on the paper? You don't need
to do them all, you can start by choosing one then
keep trying others in time.

140

My values compass

Try this when
you need a reminder
to stay grounded

You will need
Paper, markers,
coloured pencils

15 minutes

In moments of fear, you might forget the things that
keep you grounded. However, prioritizing your
values can help. Draw a compass. The four sides will
represent your strongest core values – for example,
compassion, justice, respect, and balance. Identify
which ones resonate and write them in each section.

SELF-REFLECTION Were you able to define your core
values easily, or was it difficult? Can you think of a
time when your values have helped you overcome
your fear?

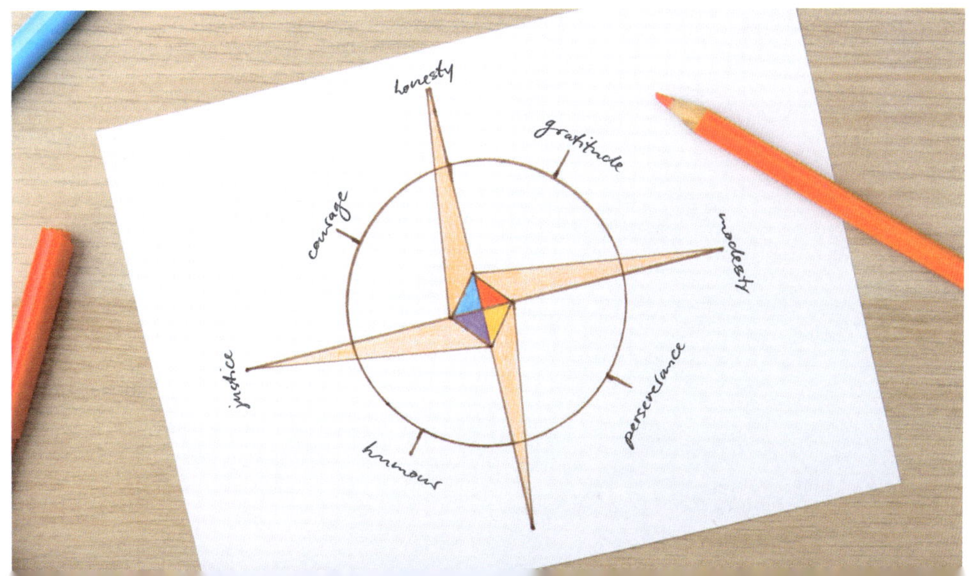

141

Courageous hero

Try this when

you want to explore what bravery means to you

You will need

Photo of someone you admire, paper, pencil, coloured pencils

20 minutes

Choose a famous person you admire for their bravery. Look online for a photo of them, then place a sheet of paper on top of the image and trace their portrait. Colour in your drawing using natural tones or as a piece of colourful abstract art. When it's complete, write down why you admire their courage.

SELF-REFLECTION Was it easy to identify someone whose courage you admire? Are they similar to you, or very different? Could their behaviours inspire you to change your own? What lessons can you learn from this person's history and apply to your own life?

142

Courageous lineage

Try this when

you need a reminder of your own strength

You will need

Paper, pencil, coloured pencils

30 minutes

Think about your family history. Who do you admire for being courageous? Draw a symbol to represent them, then write them a letter to state how much you admire them. Notice if any of the things you admire in them, you already possess. If you can, call and share your feelings with them. If you can't find a family member, then think of a friend.

SELF-REFLECTION Was it easy to identify someone you know who is brave? Is courage something that runs in your family's history? Can you find inspiration in the people around you to control your own fears?

A moment for courage

Courage isn't necessarily about heroic acts, as many people might think. It is about showing up honestly and wholeheartedly in your everyday life. Courage can help you face your fears by drawing on your values to overcome obstacles like self-doubt or being misunderstood. Whether you are standing up for what you believe in, setting boundaries, or following your childhood dreams, you can rely on this virtue to move past uncertainty. Courage isn't the absence of fear, it is about being in touch with your own vulnerability and deciding that your values are important. To build courage, you need to explore your inner world with curiosity instead of judgement. And this takes practice. Through small daily acts of bravery, you can help develop resilience and realize that you can face anything.

143

First step

Try this when
your fear is holding you back

You will need
Paper, markers, coloured pencils

15 minutes

Think of something you want to do but are afraid of attempting as it's outside your comfort zone. Put a piece of paper on the floor, then step onto it with one foot and draw around it. Inside this outline, write what personal values you would be honouring by doing the thing you are afraid of. For example, "I am doing this to fight for justice". You can highlight your values using different colours and by making the writing large or small.

SELF-REFLECTION Was it easy to identify which values are important to you? Where did you learn to appreciate these values? Can leaning into your values help motivate you to step outside your comfort zone and face your fear?

144

Second step

Try this when
you are ready to step outside your comfort zone

You will need
Paper, markers, coloured pencils

15 minutes

Put another piece of paper on the floor and draw the outline of the foot you didn't use in the previous exercise. Take a moment to acknowledge any lingering fears that arise from taking a first step outside your comfort zone, then write these around the outside of your drawing. Allow yourself to be vulnerable and acknowledge things that could be holding you back. Inside your drawing, write or draw symbols to represent the different people in your life that you can rely on to provide support when you encounter difficulties stepping outside your comfort zone.

SELF-REFLECTION Was it easy to identify who you can lean on when fear is keeping you hemmed in? Are these people aligned with your values? Sometimes, doing things with others can help us become more courageous and fight for what we want in life.

145

Holding vulnerability

Try this when
you feel vulnerable

You will need
Fragile object, pencil, markers

30 minutes

Fear can leave you feeling insecure, so look around your home for a fragile object to represent this vulnerability. Sketch this object, then imagine you are storing it safely inside a box. How would you protect it? Draw it on your page. Try to find meaning behind each protective layer. Perhaps bubble wrap represents your friends, and layers of tissue paper are your family.

SELF-REFLECTION Was it easy to find metaphorical representations of the things that protect you? How did it feel to acknowledge your vulnerability?

146

Targeting courage

Try this when
you want to celebrate your strengths

You will need
Paper, watercolours, paintbrushes, pen

30 minutes

Draw a small circle in the centre of the paper. Inside, write an affirmation that connects you with courage. For example, "I am enough", "I choose courage over comfort", or "I believe in myself". Then, draw a larger circle around it, repeating the affirmation. Draw a third circle around this and again write the affirmation. Keep going until you have a complete target. If this is uncomfortable, take some deep breaths and remind yourself that it's okay to embrace the good within you. Once the first drawing is complete, do another with a different affirmation, then continue to fill the page with more targets and affirmations.

SELF-REFLECTION Were you empowered or embarrassed by creating positive affirmations about yourself? Could this be a reflection of how comfortable you are with your own strengths? Could you use more time celebrating yourself to increase your sense of inner power and ability to face your fears?

147

Courage in vulnerability

Try this when
you are ready to embrace
your vulnerabilities

You will need
Paper, pencil, watercolours,
paintbrushes

20 minutes

Print out or draw the outline of a human body.
Try to identify where your vulnerability lives inside
your body and how you experience it, then draw
abstract shapes or colours to represent it inside the
body template. Add symbols of protection, such as
an animal you find strong or inspiring. Notice how
there is power in acknowledging your vulnerabilities
and celebrate this.

SELF-REFLECTION Was it hard or easy to sit with your
vulnerable self in this way? How did it feel to draw
protections around it? Did realizing your capacity to
defend yourself increase your self-trust and ability
to face your fears? How can becoming aware of your
own power help you protect yourself?

148

Personal shield

Try this when
you need to remember how
strong you really are

You will need
Paper, pencil, coloured pencils

20 minutes

Draw a medieval shield, then divide the inside of
the shield into four sections. In the first quadrant,
draw a symbol that represents your favourite
personal strength. In the second, draw a
representation of a core value that means the
most to you. Draw a symbol of the people that
support you in the third quadrant, and something
to represent a past experience where you showed
courage in the fourth. Keep this shield somewhere
safe, and the next time you feel scared, look at it
to reconnect with who you are and remind yourself
why you can face the fear.

SELF-REFLECTION Was it empowering to create your
own shield? What was it like to hold everything you
need to face your fears in one space? Did you notice
an improved sense of trust in your ability to face
your fears?

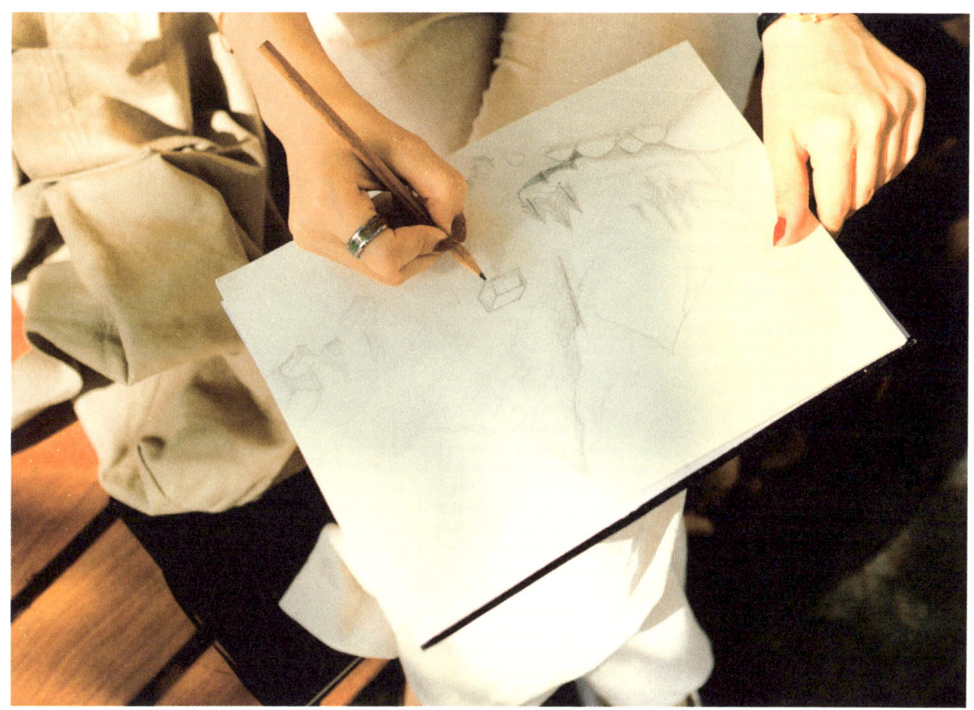

149

Rising the mountain

Try this when
you need to remember how
far you've come

You will need
Paper, pencil, coloured pencils

20 minutes

Think of a previous fear you have faced up to and
conquered, then draw a mountain. At the base of the
mountain write down where you started that journey,
and at the top, write where that journey ended for
you. Draw markers along the contours of the
mountain to represent the different lessons you
learnt along the way, and write them down.

SELF-REFLECTION Were you able to identify any
lessons you learnt as you faced your fears? Can
looking at this drawing remind you of your own
capabilities and resilience? Can you trust yourself
to rise to any fearful occasion?

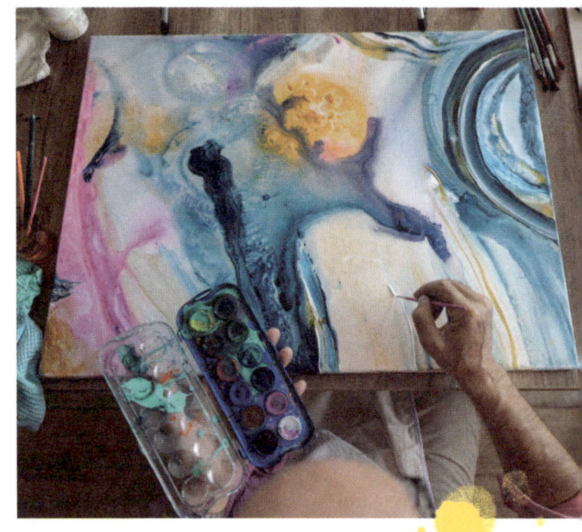

Embracing the unknown through hope

When the future feels uncertain, it's natural to experience stress, anxiety, or worry, but it's important to find healthy ways to work through this. Connecting with hope – the quiet belief that something good is still possible – can be a powerful tool. It helps alleviate apprehension and can provide the strength needed in challenging times.

150

Meet worry, stress, and anxiety

Try this when
you feel overwhelmed

You will need
Paper, pencil, coloured pencils, markers

30 minutes

Imagine your worry, stress, and anxiety are characters in a comic book, then draw them. You can use the design to highlight their underlying characteristics: is your anxiety big and strong because it causes you physical discomfort? Is stress occupying more space on the page because you are currently experiencing difficulties in your life? Write a description next to each one. What makes the character strong? What makes it weak? What does it love? What does it hate? Where does it live? Finish by naming each character.

SELF-REFLECTION What do your characters say about the way you experience worry, stress, and anxiety? Do your characters look similar, or are they very different? Why might this be? Are they scary or funny? Could this reflect how you approach your concerns about the future?

151

Where do they live?

Try this when
you feel stuck in your own head

You will need
Paper, pencil, coloured pencils, markers

10 minutes

Using the characters from the previous exercise, check in with yourself and consider where they live in your body. Draw the body part, then decorate it using representative colours and soft or sharp lines, or add specific images inside it to reflect the environment each character inhabits.

SELF-REFLECTION How does your character's space look and feel? Do they occupy a big or small area within you? Could this be a reflection of how much influence these feelings exert over you?

152

Sitting with stress

Try this when
you need to release tension

You will need
Paper, markers, timer

10 minutes

Choose a colour that represents your stress. How do you experience it? Is it making your heart beat fast? Or is it a slow and pressured sensation? Set a timer for 1 minute and move your marker across the page, following a rhythm that feels right. When the timer stops, breathe deeply for another minute. Repeat this until you feel calmer.

SELF-REFLECTION Was your movement slow or fast? Could this be an expression of how you react in times of stress? Do you become agitated, or do you freeze?

153

Worry jar part 1

Try this when
your mind won't stop racing

You will need
An empty jar,
paper, paint, pen

20+ minutes

Writing your thoughts down and questioning their validity can help you gain control over them. Decorate an empty jar with symbols and colours that represent hope, strength, and safety. Whenever a worry surfaces, write it down and put it inside the jar. Once the jar is full, empty it and start again.

SELF-REFLECTION Was it easy to identify symbols? Did writing your worries down allow you to let go of them more easily? Or did gathering them making you feel more anxious?

154

Worry jar part 2

Try this when
you want to challenge
your worries

You will need
Your worry jar, paper, pencil

20+ minutes

Take a piece of paper out of your worry jar. Draw two different scenarios where you have successfully faced this worry head-on. Try to be as imaginative as possible with solutions. If you find this exercise enjoyable, repeat it with other worries from the jar.

SELF-REFLECTION Did you find it easy or challenging to come up with multiple solutions for a single worry? Was it difficult to think imaginatively?

A moment
for anxiety

The word "anxiety" is often misunderstood – it's more than just feeling nervous or worried. Anxiety happens when your brain senses a threat, which can cause physical reactions, such as muscle tension, a racing heart, or interrupted sleep. It can be very scary, especially if your mind is warning you that something bad is about to happen. Experiencing anxiety doesn't mean there is something wrong with you. In fact, it is a natural response as your nervous system tries to protect you from potential threats. However, the problem arises when anxiety becomes overwhelming, particularly if you don't have the right coping skills. This can lead to a constant state of worry that feels impossible to switch off. If anxiety is disrupting your life, affecting your ability to work or socialize, consider seeking help from a specialist.

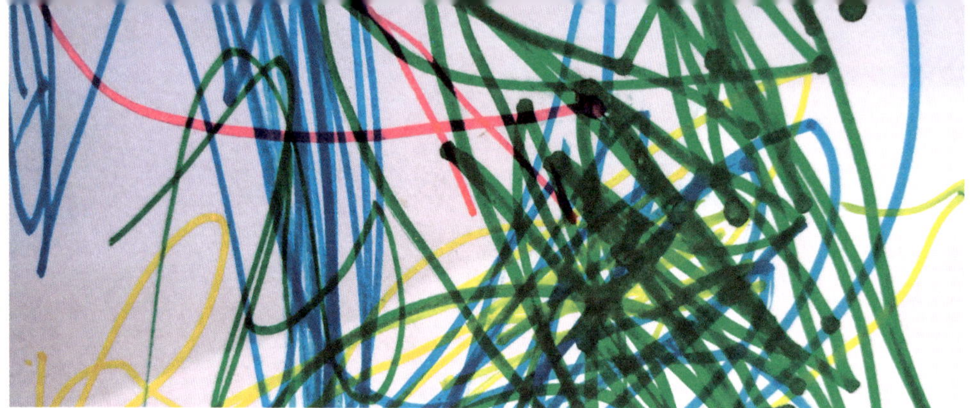

155

Intentional calm down

Try this when
you want to embrace a
slower pace of life

You will need
Paper, markers,
coloured pencils

10 minutes

Scribble very quickly on a piece of paper, adding
pressure to the marker until you have covered
most of the page. Take a moment to pause and
acknowledge how you feel, then gradually transition
into colouring in every section where the lines
intersect, going slowly and softly.

SELF-REFLECTION How did it feel to connect to a fast,
pressured pace on purpose? Did it allow space for
anxious or stressful feelings to exist? How did it feel
to slow down and release the pressure? Are there
any areas of your life where you need to become
more intentional about slowing down?

156

Release physical tension

Try this when
your body is holding
emotional tension

You will need
Paper, coloured
pencils, timer

10+ minutes

Notice where you are feeling tension in your body.
Now experiment with drawing different shapes using
circles or lines, to identify which shapes feel most
connected to this area of your body. Once you have
discovered the best one for you, set a timer for 30
seconds and draw this shape all over the page as fast
as you can. When the timer stops, take a 10-second
pause and breathe slowly. Repeat this exercise until
you feel better. You may feel tearful, and that is okay.

SELF-REFLECTION How was the experience of releasing
tension through art? Was it cathartic?

157
Inviting physical relaxation

Try this when
you want to soothe your
nervous system

You will need
Paper, coloured pencils, timer

10+ minutes

Notice where tension is stored in your
body and, as in the previous exercise,
identify if circular or linear shapes feel
most connected to this area of your body
in this moment. Once you have decided,
set a timer for 30 seconds and draw as
slowly as you can. Try to combine this
slow rhythm of drawing with your
breathing. Take a 10-second break, then
repeat the exercise and try to draw even
slower. Do this until you feel relaxed.

SELF-REFLECTION Was it comfortable or
uncomfortable to slow down? Might you
need to sit with the discomfort of the
fast-paced world first before focusing
on slowing down and relaxing?

158
This is uncertainty!

Try this when
you feel anxious about the future

You will need
Magazine or printed image, paper,
coloured pencils

20 minutes

Think of an upcoming challenge and
how it's making you feel. Then think of a
metaphorical way to represent it – maybe
you feel like a volcano about to explode.
Look for a representative image online
or in a book or magazine, and print it out
or draw it. You might want to edit this
image so that it accurately represents
how you are feeling.

SELF-REFLECTION How did it feel to
transform your words into imagery?
Was the visual representation more
accurate? Sometimes, just having a
precise portrayal of the feeling can
help liberate it and improve your
mood. Was this the case for you?

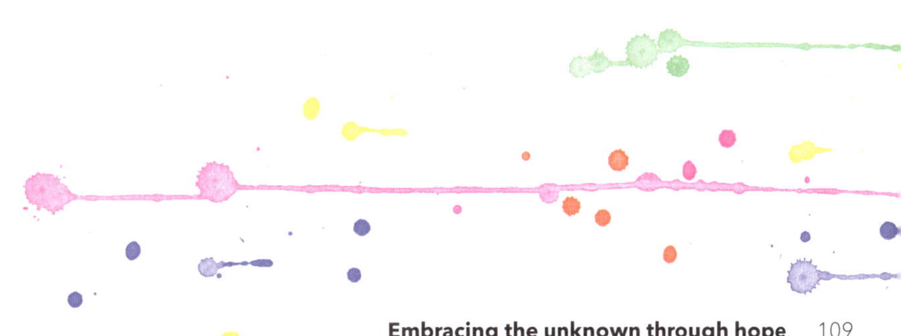

159
Uncovering the anxiety source

Try this when
you are struggling with racing thoughts

You will need
Paper, pencil, paint, paintbrushes, timer

20 minutes

Draw a torch casting a circular beam of light, and paint the background black around the lamp and illuminated area. Once complete, set a timer for 3 minutes, then close your eyes and meditate, focusing your attention on your breath. While meditating, you will notice that your mind is wandering. Try to acknowledge your thoughts before returning your attention to your breath. When the timer stops, write down all the thoughts you remember inside the light area of your drawing. Is there a pattern or string of repetitive thoughts? This could be the source of your anxiety.

SELF-REFLECTION Were you able to stay connected to your breath for extended periods of time or were you experiencing lots of disruptive thoughts? Did you notice any repetitive thoughts or patterns of thinking that could reveal what is happening inside you right now?

160
Letting go

Try this when
your thoughts are taking over

You will need
Paper, pencil, eraser

20 minutes

Draw your hand holding a bunch of balloons on strings. Inside each balloon, write down a worry or unhelpful thought. Take a moment to acknowledge these, notice any feelings that come up, and gently reflect on whether there's anything you can do to ease or address them. Then take a deep breath in, and as you exhale, erase your hand and some of the balloon strings. Now draw an open hand in its place to symbolize that you are able to let go of some of these thoughts for now.

SELF-REFLECTION Were there many thoughts you wanted to let go of? Were you able to release some of them? How did it feel to erase the hand and draw an open hand instead?

161

Stop the thought train!

Try this when
you want to put your thoughts into perspective

You will need
Paper, pencil, coloured pencils, markers, eraser

20 minutes

Draw a train made up of different cars. On each car, write down any unhelpful recurring thoughts you experience. Draw yourself as the train conductor at the front. Remember, you are the one in charge and can guide your thinking. Now take a moment to reflect. Are these thoughts true? If the answer is no, every time they show up remind yourself that they are just thoughts and you are okay. Consider what purpose these thoughts serve. If you find there is something you can do to change things, go ahead and do so. But if this isn't working, consider what you might tell a friend if they shared these thoughts with you. If it feels appropriate, erase the thoughts.

SELF-REFLECTION Were you able to identify your repetitive thoughts? How was the experience of seeing them written down? Were they realistic concerns or imaginary worries?

162

Transforming anxious thoughts

Try this when
you feel overwhelmed by other people's problems

You will need
Paper, pencil, coloured pencils, pen

20 minutes

Sometimes, trying to control situations that are beyond your circle of influence can lead to anxiety. To recognize that this feeling is usually related to problems that you can't change, it's important to identify them. Write down your worries, then on another piece of paper, trace the outline of your hand. Try to write which problems you don't have control over around the outline of your hand, such as how others think or what they do. Inside the hand, write down the problems that you do have control over, such as how *you* react and your feelings.

SELF-REFLECTION Was it difficult to differentiate between problems that belong to you and which problems don't? Could your worries be related to other people's problems, thoughts, or feelings?

163

Bin the thought

Try this when
you want to let go of thoughts
that no longer serve you

You will need
Paper, pen, scissors

15 minutes

Using the free-style writing technique
(p.90), write down all your thoughts
until you fill three pages. Remember,
you can write whatever comes to mind.
Once done, identify the thoughts that
you want to change, cut them out, and
rewrite them on another piece of paper
by re-framing them as something
positive, optimistic, or kinder for you.
When you've finished, throw any
thoughts away that aren't needed any
more and say goodbye to them.

SELF-REFLECTION Was it easy or hard to sit
with your own thoughts? How did it feel
to deconstruct your own train of thought
and to cut out thoughts? Was rewriting
your thoughts a positive experience?

164

Tap the stress away

Try this when
you want to release stress

You will need
Paper, paint

15 minutes

Instead of bottling up your worries,
use finger painting to release some of
the accumulated energy. Choose one to
three colours to represent your stress or
anxiety, then paint a sheet of paper using
your fingertips and a tapping movement,
similar to playing the piano or typing.
Play with speed. First go as fast as you
can, then use slow movements.

SELF-REFLECTION Was the sensory
experience of the paint pleasant or
uncomfortable for you? Sometimes,
physical movement can increase
emotional expression and be cathartic.
Which speed felt more aligned with
your stress or anxiety? Could this be a
sign you need to speed things up for
yourself, or should you slow down?

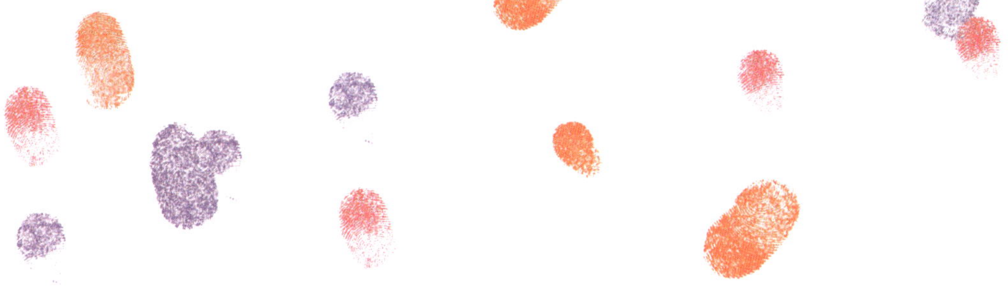

165

Glimmer of hope

Try this when
the future feels scary

You will need
Paper, pencil, coloured pencils

15 minutes

Draw three candles, then colour them in using colours that represent hope for you. On one of the candles, write the name of someone who can help ignite your own hope, such as a positive friend or family member who provides comfort and wisdom. On the second candle, write down personal strengths you have used in the past to deal with hardship. For example, could your determination or creativity be helpful to face your fears? On the third one, write down a small action you can take to feel better, such as journalling or going for a walk in nature.

SELF-REFLECTION Were you able to find ideas for the three candles? Did you notice how there are things within your control in the present moment that can help ease your worries?

166

Ray of hope

Try this when
you want to feel more hopeful about what's ahead

You will need
Paper, watercolours, paintbrushes

20 minutes

Draw a cloudy sky in a landscape of your choice, then paint rays of light breaking through the clouds and shining on the land. On each of the rays, write down things that give you hope for the future.

SELF-REFLECTION Were you able to think of things that spark optimism? How did it feel to see them through a landscape? Can the beauty of nature be a reminder of hope on its own?

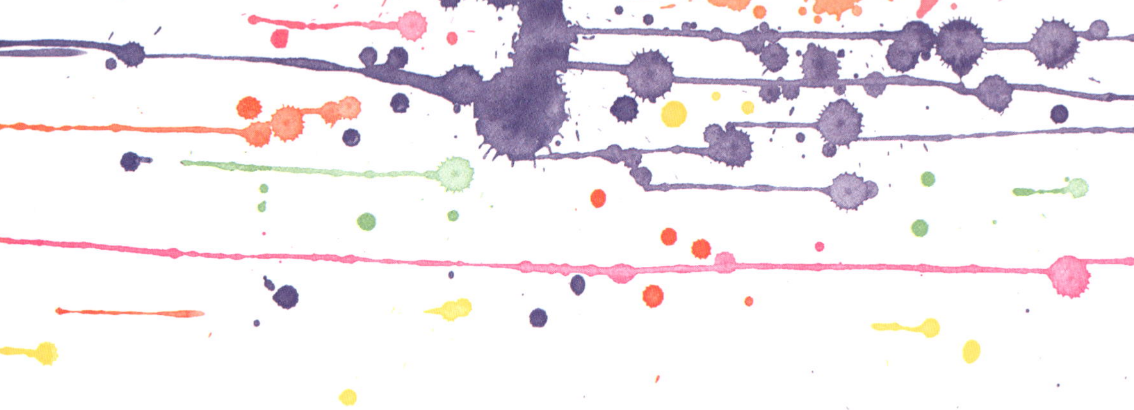

167

Bucket of hope

Try this when
you want to feel more
positive about the future

You will need
Box, pen, paper

20+ minutes

Find a box or container where you can store your
ideas. For the next two weeks, write down at least
one thing each day that gives you faith in the future.
Maybe you saw someone helping a stranger, or
flowers blooming from the cracks on a city street.
Look for hope around you. At the end of the two
weeks, empty the box and read through everything.

SELF-REFLECTION Was it difficult to find hope in
humanity? Could this be a sign you have been
surrounded by constant negativity recently? Are
there other ways you can foster positive feelings
for the future?

168

Tree of hope

Try this when
you need a boost of hope

You will need
Paper, pencil, markers,
watercolours, coloured
pencils

25 minutes

Draw your favourite tree as a representation of
yourself. Draw strong roots coming from it, then
inside the roots write down personal affirmations,
such as "I find solutions" and "I am protected". Inside
the trunk, write down examples of past experiences
you have overcome, then on the branches, write your
dreams and aspirations for the future.

SELF-REFLECTION Were you able to recognize your
ability to face challenges? Did this make you feel
more optimistic about the future?

169

The four seasons of hope

Try this when
you are ready to embrace
new beginnings

You will need
Paper, pencil, markers,
watercolours, paintbrushes,
coloured pencils

15 minutes

Use the same tree you drew in the previous exercise, but this time, draw four versions to represent it changing through the seasons. Under the spring tree, write about a moment when you were excited about a future project. Under the summer one, write a story about when you successfully achieved what you wanted. Under the autumn tree, write about when you had to let go of something. Use the winter tree to reflect on when stopping and resting was necessary before continuing a challenging journey. Once complete, think about how just like trees, we have seasons within our own lives, and ending one thing will become a new beginning.

SELF-REFLECTION Have you noticed seasons in your own life? Can you use this metaphor to allow yourself to get comfortable with things coming to an end?

170

Looking for hope

Try this when
you need to smile

You will need
Paper, art materials you
find comfortable

25 minutes

Search online for some good news. Find reports that are uplifting or inspirational for you. Choose three different stories, then, using materials you feel most comfortable with, draw and colour in an image that represents each of them.

SELF-REFLECTION How was the experience of purely reading articles about good news? Did it feel strange or satisfying? Could this be a reflection of your news consumption patterns and a sign that you need to change some of them? Were you able to find good news that made you smile?

171

I can do this!

Try this when
you feel overwhelmed
about the future

You will need
Paper, pen

15 minutes

Think of a problem that is making you feel worried, stressed, or anxious. Consider what skills you need to face these challenges, then imagine that you are creating a CV to apply for the job of fixing the problem. Highlight which skills and abilities you possess that could help you. Think about any past experiences where you have resolved issues, and which tools, personal lessons, or networks you used to make things right. Write them down.

SELF-REFLECTION Did you find it easy to apply for the job? Were you able to identify the skills that can help you solve your own problems? Are there areas that you still need to work on or add to your CV?

172

Rising above challenges

Try this when
you doubt yourself

You will need
Paper, black marker, yellow paint, paintbrush, pen

25 minutes

Using a black marker, cover a page with scribbles that express your feelings of worry, stress, or anxiety. Take a moment, then paint yellow hearts on top of the scribbles and allow them to dry. Using a pen, write positive affirmations such as "I can do this", "I am strong", and "I am creative" inside the hearts.

SELF-REFLECTION Did you enjoy the process of layering both negative and positive on the same page? Was it easy or difficult to find positive affirmations? Could this be related to your ability of trusting yourself when faced with a challenge?

173

Shine your light

Try this when
you need to see your
positive impact

You will need
Paper, black marker, yellow
paint, paintbrush, pen

25 minutes

Draw a light source with the light shining from it.
It could be a table lamp, a lantern, or a lighthouse.
In the glowing light, write the different ways in which
you give hope to others.

SELF-REFLECTION What source of light did you draw?
Was it small or big? Could this reflect how you see
yourself and your ability to positively influence
others? Have you noticed how giving other people
hope can make you feel better and more uplifted?

174

A better world

Try this when
you want to imagine
a brighter future

You will need
Paper, favourite materials

30 minutes

Using any materials of your choice, create an
imaginary world that is better than the one you live
in. Notice what makes it special or different. Take a
moment to reflect on how you could help make this
utopia a reality.

SELF-REFLECTION Was your version of a better world
very different from your current world or was it
similar? Could you identify small steps you can take
to help make your world a better place?

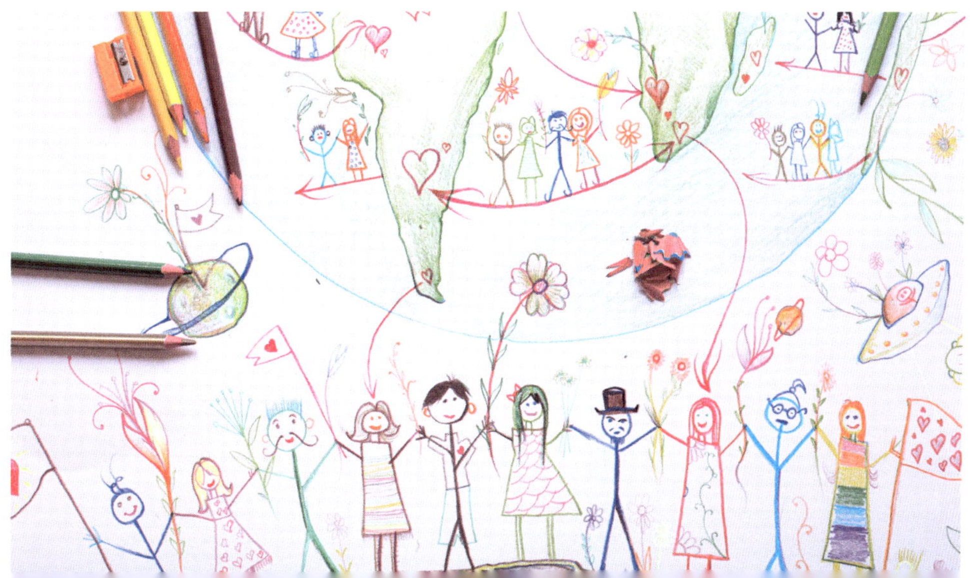

Be inspired

When you feel lost, hope can help you find the force within to navigate a way out. This source of light is all around you – you just have to take the time to connect with it. Let art be your guide.

Try this when
you want to feel more hopeful

4 hours

175 **Reignite your spark**

You will need
Markers, sticky notes

Watch an uplifting film that gives you faith in the future. On sticky notes, write down some quotes from the film that inspire you. Place them somewhere visible as a reminder.

176 **Let hope guide you**

You will need
Paper, pencil, coloured pencils, markers, watercolours, paintbrushes

Look around for art that signifies hope. It might include light and warm colours, and optimistic themes or symbols such as sunrises and birds. Search online or in books, or visit a gallery. Choose a piece that resonates with you, then try to recreate it, tweaking it to your liking.

177 **Awaken your inner power**

You will need

Paper, watercolours, paintbrushes

Paint a sun that nearly fills an entire sheet of paper. Let it dry, then write the lyrics of a song that makes you feel strong on top of it. You can listen to the song while you paint, if you wish.

SELF-REFLECTION Did you choose a film you already knew, or was it one you haven't seen before? Can you relate to any particular character? If so, why? What called your attention to the artwork you chose? Did recreating the art change your perspective of the piece? Was the song you selected from your past or something current? Could this relate to where your source of hope can come from?

178

My little light

Try this when
life feels heavy

You will need
Empty jar, coloured tissue
paper, glue, water, paintbrush,
candle

20+ minutes

Choose some tissue paper in colours that feel
connected to hope. These can be light, warm, or
vibrant tones – whatever feels right to you. Cut
the paper into shapes or symbols that represent
hope for you, then glue these around the outside
of your jar. As you work, think of something that
reminds you that your future can be bright. This
might be a memory, a person, a place, or simply
the possibility of change. Let your jar dry, then fix a
small candle inside as a symbol of this light, to guide
you when times feel dark.

SELF-REFLECTION When was the last time you felt
hopeful? What does your jar reveal to you about your
own sources of hope? Where in your life could this
light be invited in?

179

Abstract hope

Try this when
you want to connect
with hope

You will need
Paper, pencil, coloured
pencils, markers

15+ minutes

Think of colours that represent hope for you, then
colour in a piece of paper with them. Draw symbols
or shapes that represent hope for you on top – these
could be stars, rainbows, spirals, or hearts.

SELF-REFLECTION How did it feel to connect with hope
intentionally? Did creating something abstract make
it easier to tap into the feeling, or do you prefer more
realistic, concrete representations?

180
Becoming hope

Try this when
you need a pick-me-up

You will need
Your wardrobe

15+ minutes

Choose three colours that represent hope for you, then go to your wardrobe and find articles of clothing in similar shades. Wear them on days when you feel worried about the future and use them as a reminder that things can work out in your favour.

SELF-REFLECTION Was the colour palette you chose a surprise? Did you have several pieces in your wardrobe in the colours you chose? When wearing these clothes, could you connect with your intention to feel hopeful?

181
Hope path

Try this when
you need to remember that things will be okay in the end

You will need
Paper, markers, coloured pencils

15+ minutes

Think of a time when hope helped you overcome a difficult period. Draw a path showing what that journey looked like. Add drawings to represent where hope helped you keep going. Maybe a loved one, song, or life event reminded you that everything was going to be okay. Use these symbols as a reminder to look out for them in your life now.

SELF-REFLECTION Are you naturally optimistic when it comes to facing obstacles? What helped you hold on to hope in the past? Was it connecting with others, or was it the arts, or a mixture of both?

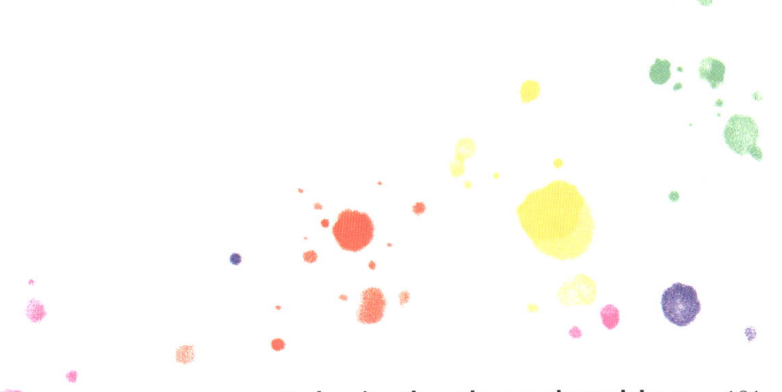

Letting go of anger, inviting calm

Anger is a powerful emotion. It is a natural response to moments when your boundaries are crossed, or are close to being crossed. However, many of us were never taught how to express it in a healthy way, so we bottle it up until we explode. To improve your relationship with this feeling and so achieve better outcomes for your health, you need to learn to acknowledge and explore it with curiosity.

182
Meet anger

Try this when
you want to explore your
relationship with anger

You will need
Paper, magazine or image
printouts, scissors, glue,
markers, coloured pencils

30 minutes

Before learning to manage anger, you need
to understand how you relate to this emotion.
Create a collage about how you experience anger
in your life. Find images of people that you perceive
as angry and choose those who you feel represent
your behaviour when angered. Think about how you
handle yourself when provoked.

SELF-REFLECTION Do you have a comfortable
relationship with your anger? Or is it complicated?
Are you confrontational or avoidant? Do you feel
empowered, or are you afraid of yourself?

183
Anger in my
social systems

Try this when
anger feels like
someone else's voice

You will need
Paper, markers,
coloured pencils

25 minutes

How you relate to your anger is probably connected
to how your family and/or close social circles have
talked about it and acted on it. Draw how your
different family members or others close to you
express their anger.

SELF-REFLECTION Did you grow up with the freedom
to express your anger? Was this feeling used to cover
up other emotions, such as sadness or fear? How did
others influence your ability to connect with this
emotion? Did you find any patterns in the drawing
that you recognize in yourself?

Hello! My name is anger

In order to manage your anger, you need to first understand it better. Taking the time to notice how anger shows up for you makes you more mindful of this feeling and reduces your risk of reacting impulsively. This powerful emotion can feel either threatening or empowering, so owning its narrative is important to go from being controlled by it to being in control of it.

Try this when
you want to take control of your anger
1 hour 40 minutes

184 Introducing anger

You will need
Paper, markers, coloured pencils

Externalizing your anger can help you see it through a different lens and have more control over it. First, draw a character that represents your anger, then write down its characteristics, including strengths, weaknesses, and unique traits. Think about what makes your anger more powerful or weaker, and if it prefers to be called a certain name. Observe how this character is different from those you have created before.

185 What are you doing, anger?

You will need
Paper, markers, coloured pencils

Next, draw a comic book strip where your character interacts with happiness, fear, and sadness. Does it treat happiness with respect? Is it fair when dealing with fear? How is its relationship with sadness? Does your character overpower or protect others?

186 **How can we be friends?**

You will need

Paper, markers,
coloured pencils

Now, draw another comic book strip featuring your anger character, but this time imagine it interacting with the same three emotions from the previous exercise in a different way. Allow yourself freedom to depict how you wish your anger would treat others.

187 **Interviewing anger**

You will need

Paper, pencil,
coloured pencils,
markers

When you feel angry, connect with your anger character to try to uncover the cause. Place it in front of you and, using the free-writing technique (p.90), answer the following questions, filling a page for each: why are you here today? What do you need from me? What are you protecting me from? Read through your answers and notice if there are any themes or patterns emerging that can help you understand your anger.

SELF-REFLECTION Did you find it difficult to create this character? Do you like it, or do you feel afraid of it? Could this reflect your relationship with your anger? What can you identify from the interactions with other feelings? Does this relate to your experience of anger in your own life? Could you benefit from allowing other emotions to step in? Could the changes you drew in the second-to-last exercise be implemented when dealing with your anger? Were there any responses that surprised you? Could there be something you're ignoring that your character wants acknowledged? Can you see your anger as a protector, or does it feel like an enemy?

188

The pressure gauge

Try this when
you want to explore the
intensity of your anger

You will need
Paper, markers,
coloured pencils

15 minutes

Draw a pressure gauge to represent your anger.
Mark the different levels of anger you experience,
from calm, frustrated, irritated, and upset to angry,
furious, and enraged. Notice where your needle
usually points to.

SELF-REFLECTION Were you aware of the different
degrees of anger? Is there a particular intensity of
anger you tend to gravitate towards? How would it
be to allow yourself to experience the full range of
feelings of anger?

189

My anger triggers

Try this when
you need to prevent
anger outbursts

You will need
Paper, coloured pencils

15 minutes

In the centre of a piece of paper, write "I feel angry
when…" Surround this phrase with at least three
drawings of scenarios that represent situations that
may trigger feelings of anger.

SELF-REFLECTION Was it difficult to identify things that
make you angry? If you struggled to identify your
triggers, why might that be? If this was easy and you
thought of multiple scenarios, could it be that anger
is a comfortable feeling and masks other emotions?

190

The calm after
the storm

Try this when
you want to explore how
anger shapes your life

You will need
Paper, coloured pencils

30 minutes

Divide a piece of paper in half. On one side, draw
a shoreline where a storm, inspired by your anger,
is erupting. On the other side, create the same
shoreline after the storm. Notice the differences.

SELF-REFLECTION How bad was the storm you
created? Is this how you experience your anger?
Is it scary? Was the second drawing heavily impacted
by the storm, or is it looking clean, as if nothing had
happened? Could this be a reflection of how you
wish life could be without anger?

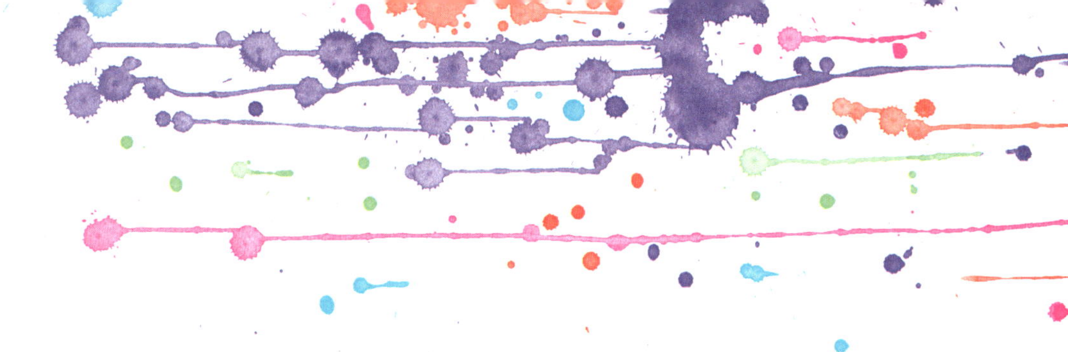

191

Tear and repair

Try this when
you want to make
space for your anger

You will need
Paper, coloured pencils, watercolours,
paintbrushes, scissors, glue

30 minutes

Anger is a feeling that can connect
you with aggression and a need for
destruction. Express your anger on the
top of the page. It can be a scribble,
symbol, or you can fill the paper with
an angry colour. Then tear this paper into
pieces. You can scream while you do this
if it feels right and it's appropriate for the
space you are in. When you are done,
create a collage with the torn pieces.

SELF-REFLECTION How did it feel
to destroy something on purpose?
Were you able to find a sense of relief?
Allowing space for destruction can be
necessary when anger is overpowering
you. In comparison, how did it feel to
put the pieces together again?

192

Smash and sculpt

Try this when
you need a healthy way
to express your anger

You will need
Clay or Play-Doh, timer

10+ minutes

Anger creates a lot of energy, so
releasing it in a contained manner can
make it easier to let go of the feeling.
Channel your anger by pounding clay
for 5 minutes – smash it, roll it, squeeze
it as hard as you can, break it apart, or
throw it to the ground to release tension.
Once you feel that your stuck energy
has gone, take a moment to pause and
breathe, then slowly reshape the clay
into a calm symbol or sculpture.

SELF-REFLECTION Did using movement
and material resistance help transform
your angry energy? What was it like to
slow down and turn your anger into
something constructive? Do you think
you might be able to do the same next
time you feel angry?

193

Anger letters part 1

Try this when
you need to share your
anger safely

You will need
Favourite materials

30 minutes

Create an artwork that shows how your anger looks
to the person you are angry with. It can be a painting,
a drawing, or a scribble. Use the image as inspiration
for writing a letter to that person, explaining all the
details of your creation. Allow your anger to be fully
expressed on the page. When finished, destroy the
letter but keep the artwork for the next exercise.

SELF-REFLECTION How did it feel to express your anger
indirectly? Was it enough to let it go? If you feel the
need to discuss your feelings with the person, you
might want to share the art with them, not the letter.
Sometimes, seeing a feeling represented instead
of hearing about it in words can open deeper
conversations. Be careful, and only do it if it feels
safe for you and the other person.

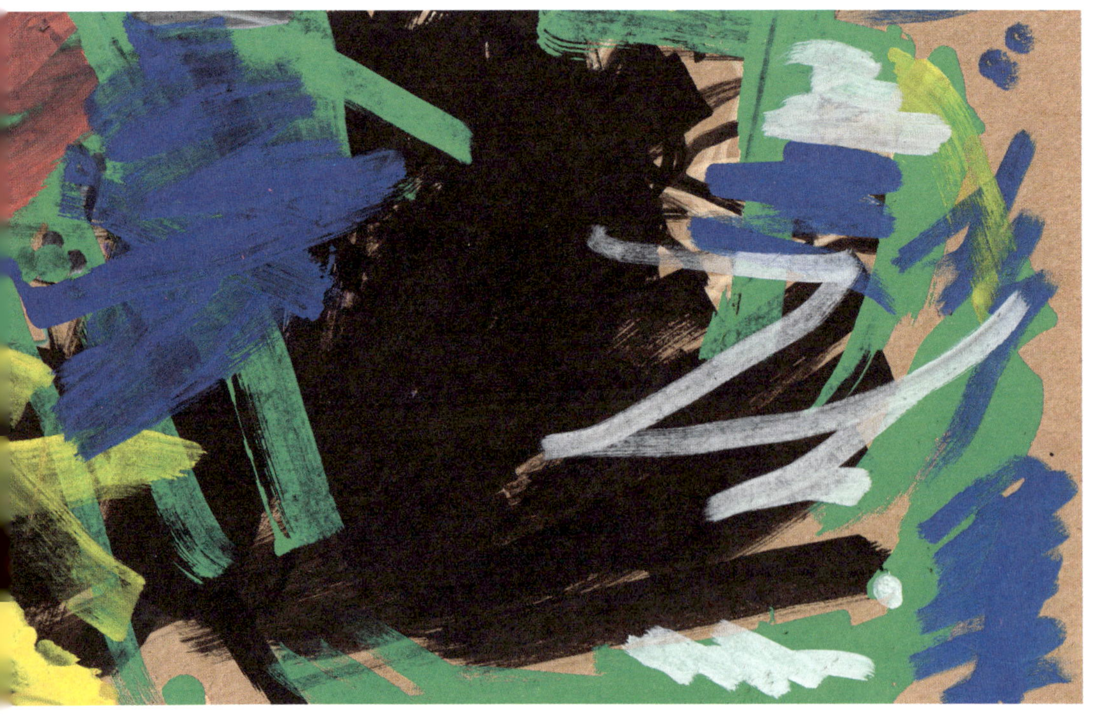

194

Anger letters part 2

Try this when
you want to listen deeply
to your anger

You will need
Previous artwork, paper,
markers, coloured pencils

20 minutes

Place the artwork from the previous exercise in front of you and imagine having a conversation with it. Start a conversation with the artwork, asking the following questions: why are you here today? What message do I need to hear about my anger? Do you have any wisdom that can help me navigate this angry feeling? Allow the imaginary dialogue to exist and don't judge it; simply take note of the information. When you've finished, write a letter to yourself reflecting on this dialogue.

SELF-REFLECTION Were you able to have a dialogue with your art, or did it feel silly? What insight from this dialogue can help you understand or manage your anger differently?

195

Silent protest

Try this when
you want to channel anger
into meaningful action

You will need
Paper, pencil, markers

15 minutes

Sometimes you need to express your anger towards injustices or in support of things that matter to you. Imagine something in the world that makes you angry. Draw yourself holding a sign that you would use to protest about the issue. Decorate it, making it as serious or as fun as you want.

SELF-REFLECTION Is your protest about a matter that you are already engaged in, or is it new? How did it feel to turn an idea into action? Feeling helpless can be a trigger for anger, so try to then use that energy for something productive instead of allowing it to consume you.

196
Alchemizing anger part 1

Try this when
you need to release bottled-up anger

You will need
Pillow

10+ minutes

Take a moment to connect with your body and notice where your anger is stored. Once you identify it, imagine a colour that represents that area. Take a pillow and start hitting it or scream into it. Imagine the colour leaving your body and being released into the atmosphere. Notice if the colour changes while you are doing this or if the emotion moves to different places in your body. Repeat until you feel that the energy has been released.

SELF-REFLECTION Did your anger stay in one part of your body, or did it shift? Could this mean that your anger is multilayered and more complex than you think? Could this anger have been stored for a while?

197
Alchemizing anger part 2

Try this when
you want to find wisdom within your anger

You will need
Paper, watercolours, paintbrushes

20 minutes

Paint a bonfire using shades of the colour you envisioned in the previous exercise. It doesn't matter if the colours are not the same as a traditional fire. If it feels safe, close your eyes, or simply look down, and imagine you are sitting by that fire when a wise person appears before you. Ask them where this anger has come from and what it needs from you. Thank them for their wisdom and, if you feel the need, write down any messages you gleaned from this exercise.

SELF-REFLECTION What did you notice about your bonfire? Was it big or small? Does this give you an idea of how big your anger is? Were you able to connect and speak to an imaginary being, or did it feel silly? Remember to open yourself up to experiencing your feelings in new ways. Was the message useful? Did it reveal any potential underlying feelings?

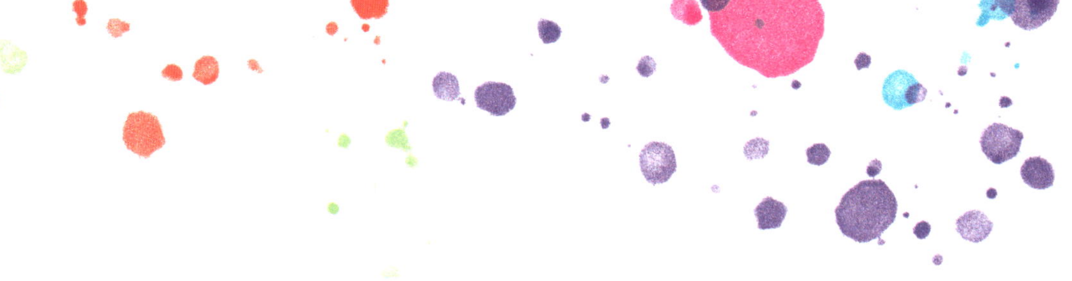

198

Angry art world part 1

Try this when
your anger makes you feel alone

You will need
Paper, pencil, computer or phone

15 minutes

Search online for "angry art" images until you find one that you feel represents your current experience of anger. Take a moment to connect with this art, then write down why you chose it. What do you think the artist was trying to share with the viewer? How do you think the artist was feeling when they created this piece? What emotions does this art evoke within you?

SELF-REFLECTION Was it a positive experience to see someone else's expression of anger? Did it help you to feel understood? Could your answers about the artist reflect your own emotional experience? Remember that you are not alone in challenging times.

199

Angry art world part 2

Try this when
you want to see your anger differently

You will need
Paper, materials of your choice

20 minutes

Try to recreate the image you chose in the previous exercise. The art doesn't have to look exactly the same. Imitating other people's art can help us compare and understand our own emotions better. If you feel the need to change some things to make it more personal and curated to your own emotional experience, feel free to do so.

SELF-REFLECTION Did you create the same image, or did it shift? Did changing any parts of the image help you to make it more meaningful? Did this process help you express your anger? Did you feel a sense of release once you had finished your creation? Taking inspiration from others can be liberating.

200
Boundary map

Try this when
you need to explore your
personal boundaries

You will need
Paper, markers,
coloured pencils

20 minutes

Draw a symbol that represents you in the centre of
a piece of paper. Around it, draw four large circles
labelled Physical, Emotional, Mental, and Time – these
represent the four different types of boundaries.
Inside each circle, depict how you currently see
yourself in that area. Do you feel disconnected or
overstimulated? Can you emotionally support others
right now, or are you drained? How heavy is your
mental load? Do you have free time, or is your time
very limited? Whenever you feel anger rising, pause
and check in with these boundaries before reacting.

SELF-REFLECTION How often do you check in with
your own capacities and limits? Your boundaries
constantly change. Do you respect your own
boundaries, or do you tend to push yourself to
accommodate others?

201
Protecting the castle

Try this when
you want to reflect on your
emotional defences

You will need
Paper, markers,
coloured pencils

30 minutes

Draw a castle, then draw different ways you might
protect it. When you've finished, analyse how
effective your defences are. Are they too strong,
or maybe not sufficient?

SELF-REFLECTION Could strong defences mean
you are too guarded and your anger is getting
out of control? Could weak defences mean that you
are not able to appropriately channel anger in order
to protect yourself?

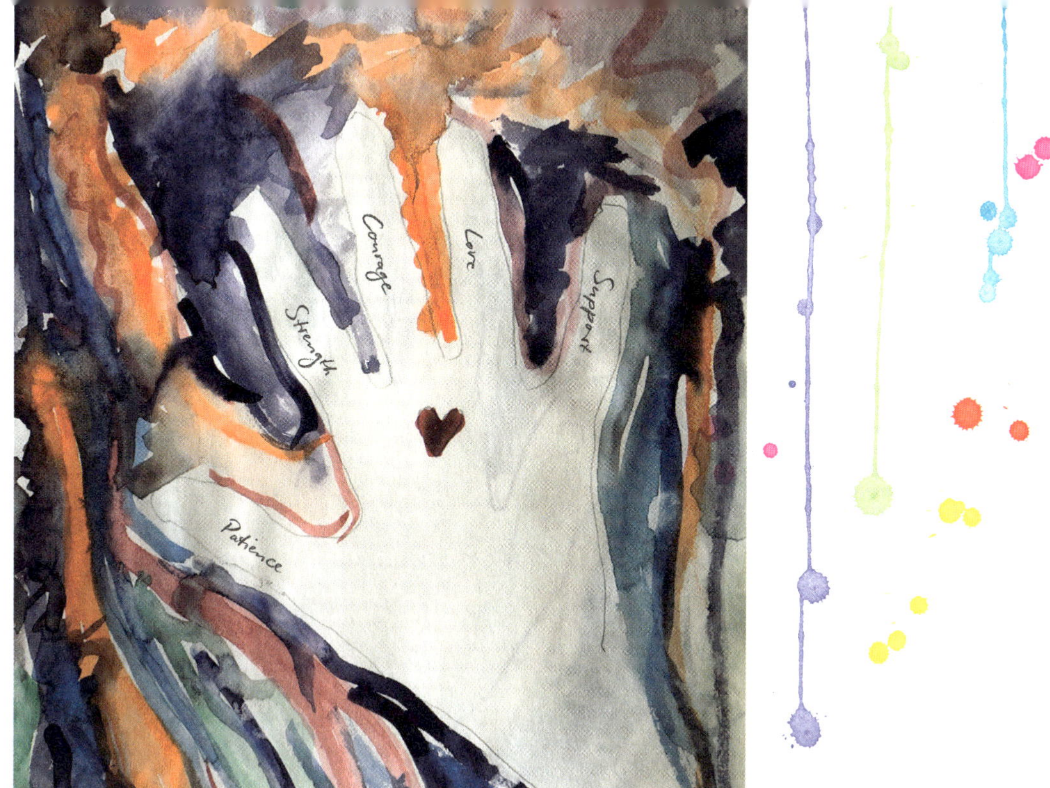

202
Yes and no hands

Try this when
you want to set clearer boundaries with others

You will need
Paper, pencil, watercolours, paintbrush

20 minutes

Use this exercise to gain clarity about the boundaries you need to set with others. Start by tracing the outlines of both your hands. Inside one hand, write what you want to invite more of into your life. In the other hand, write down the things you are no longer willing to tolerate from others – behaviours or situations that make you feel disrespected or drained. Paint the space around the hands choosing colours that reflect the emotions that come up for you.

SELF-REFLECTION Were you able to identify which boundaries are being crossed for you right now? Are there boundaries you can actively set, or are they out of your control? Could your anger be a result of these boundaries being compromised?

203

Count to 10

Try this when
you need a soothing way to
interrupt angry impulses

You will need
Paper, paint, paintbrushes

15+ minutes

The well-known exercise of counting to ten in order
to calm down is effective because it can help you
slow down and take stock before you fall prey to
angry impulses. Using a colour that is soothing for
you, paint from one side of a piece of paper to the
other using interconnecting lines, waves, or circles,
while counting slowly to 10. Repeat until the page is
full or you feel calmer.

SELF-REFLECTION Did focusing both on the painting
process and counting help calm you down? How did
it feel to paint slowly and follow a rhythm?

204

"I" statements

Try this when
you want to communicate
your anger constructively

You will need
Paper, coloured pencils

15+ minutes

Breached boundaries can cause anger, but instead
of reacting, you can learn to communicate assertively.
This means finding ways to express your thoughts
and feelings in a manner that is clear and respectful.
Assertive communication requires you to shift to
"I" statements in order to express your personal
boundaries and needs. Write down the following
phrases and fill in the blanks accordingly.

"I FEEL"
[draw an emoji face that shows how you are feeling]

"WHEN YOU"
[summarize an action that angers you]
"BECAUSE"
[define the source of your feeling]
"WHAT I NEED FROM YOU IS"
[draw what you want to see happen, regardless of
the outcome]

SELF-REFLECTION Are you used to communicating
your needs through explaining your feelings?
If not, how could you see this changing the way
you engage with people close to you?

205

Turning anger into assertiveness

Try this when
you want to practise
handling conflict calmly

You will need
Paper, pencil, coloured
pencils, markers

20+ minutes

Assertive communication is a skill that needs practice. Consider someone with whom you have had a disagreement and would like to discuss the matter. Make sure you choose a situation that isn't too triggering for you right now. This conversation is imaginary as it's a practice exercise. Create a comic strip depicting yourself and the other person, and in the first scene draw the situation that angered you. You can include thought and dialogue bubbles. In the next scene, draw yourself having a conversation with the person. Refer to the previous "I" statement exercise for inspiration. When you are drawing, be intentional about the body language your character is exhibiting, such as whether they are making eye contact, standing tall, or looking confident and calm.

SELF-REFLECTION How did it feel to have an imaginary conversation? Were you able to identify your needs and feelings and explain them in a thought bubble?

206

Soothing spirals

Try this when
you need to calm
your nervous system

You will need
Paper, coloured pencils

15+ minutes

Choose five colours that represent calm for you. Using one colour, slowly draw a spiral, starting in the centre of the page and going outwards, while repeating the phrase "Releasing anger". Change the colour and draw the same spiral, but begin at the edges and go inwards. As you do this, say, "Inviting peace in". Repeat the exercise 10 times, alternating the colours.

SELF-REFLECTION Were you able to soothe yourself through art? What was more useful – the phrases or the movement? Could this mean that you can use slow movements to calm yourself when you are feeling angry? Do you prefer auditory reminders, or a combination of words and movement?

207

Calming senses

Try this when
you want to ground yourself

You will need
Paper, pencil,
coloured pencils

20+ minutes

Go outside and find a space where you can draw in peace. Look for something colourful and draw it on a sheet of paper. If possible, listen for a sound and sketch whatever is creating that sound. It could be a waterfall, a bird, or rustling leaves. Search for a smell and draw the source. Then touch something that catches your eye and capture it with your pencil. If possible, end with something you can taste and depict it on the page.

SELF-REFLECTION How did it feel to use your senses to regain control of yourself? Were you able to use all your senses for this exercise?

NOTE If you are someone who experiences sensory differences or limitations, then focus on one sense and find five things to represent it.

208

My calm place

Try this when
you need to disconnect
from reality for a while

You will need
Paper, coloured pencils

15+ minutes

Think of a place that brings you calm and draw it. Take a moment to imagine yourself walking through this environment. Notice the smells, the temperature, the sounds, and the colours.

SELF-REFLECTION Did you create an imaginary landscape, or was it somewhere you have previously been that brings you peace? If this place exists, are able to you visit it frequently? If not, remember that you can always take a break during the day and visit it in your imagination.

A moment for mindfulness

Mindfulness is about being aware of what is happening within you and around you without judgement. It is a practice that focuses on allowing your thoughts and feelings to exist just as they are. This form of radical self-acceptance is not about relaxing, as many people might think; it's about having a different attitude towards yourself that allows you to channel calm. When you integrate mindfulness into your everyday life, you are not meditating to leave your mind in a blank state, you are training yourself to be more in control of your attention during challenging times and balancing your inner and outer worlds.

You can learn to give space to your emotions and become aware of what you need from those around you. Mindfulness improves your ability to pause before reacting and be more intentional about how you want to respond and behave.

209

You are protected part 1

Try this when
you need to remember
that you are safe

You will need
Paper, watercolours,
paintbrushes, marker

15+ minutes

When anger dominates, it might trigger
feelings of unsafety and defensiveness.
This is why you need to restore your
sense of personal security to calm down.
Either draw a human figure with a marker
or print one out, then draw a calm face
on it. Using watercolours, surround it
with a layer of soothing colours while
repeating the phrases "You are safe",
"You are protected", and "You are calm".

SELF-REFLECTION What colours did you
choose, and why were they soothing for
you? Did you feel more protected after
focusing on surrounding your drawing
with calming colours and reciting
good intentions?

210

You are protected part 2

Try this when
you are seeking comfort

You will need
Paper, watercolours,
paintbrushes, marker

15+ minutes

Once your previous creation is dry, draw
symbols over the top of it to represent
the things or behaviours that can give
this human figure safety and support.
It could be nurturing hands, a blanket,
or box cocooning the figure, or a lantern
providing a guiding light. You might
include comforting symbols such as
hearts or mandalas.

SELF-REFLECTION What symbols, ideas, or
behaviours did you identify? Were there
many, or did you struggle to find them?
How can you connect with these symbols
more often?

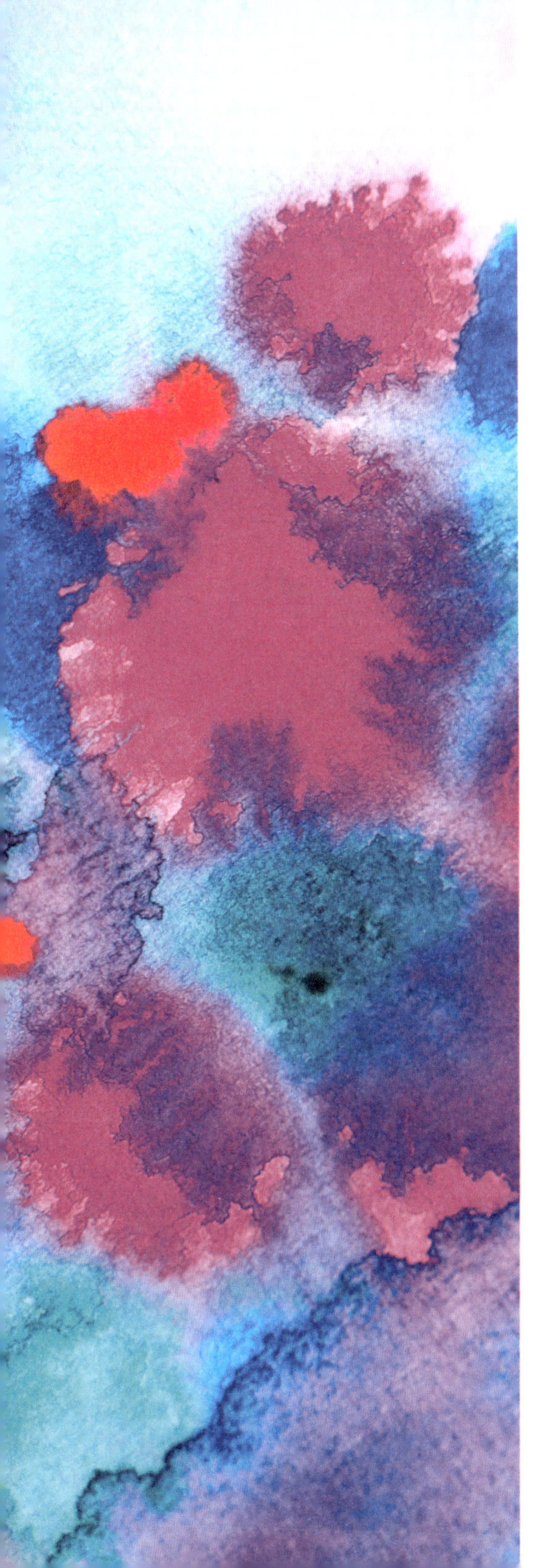

211

Reverse colouring

Try this when
you need to connect with calm

You will need
Paper, watercolours,
paintbrushes, pen, timer

20+ minutes

Connecting with the present moment is
crucial when fostering feelings of calm.
Wet a piece of paper, then fill the page
with three colours that represent calm.
Give your full attention to blending the
colours. You can sprinkle salt on top
to create different effects before letting
it dry. Once dry, set the timer for 10
minutes and use a pen to highlight all
the different things that stand out for
you. They can be recognizable figures
or abstract circles and lines.

SELF-REFLECTION Was it easy to be
present for 10 minutes, or did your mind
wander? Did any recognizable figures
emerge from your creation? Could these
symbols have a hidden message for you?

Soothing sadness, nurturing joy

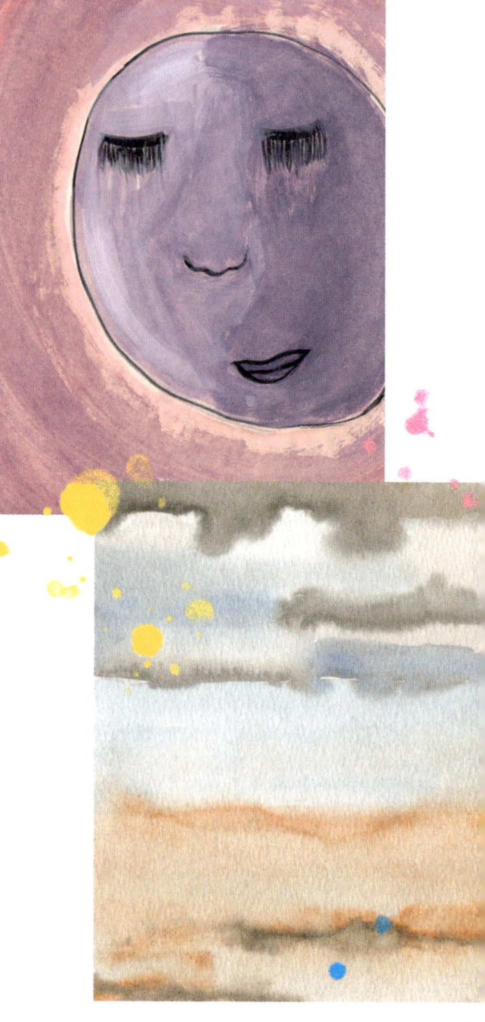

Sadness is part of being human, and is a natural response to loss, disappointment, and loneliness. However, we often try to avoid this emotion because of the heaviness it brings and the sense of vulnerability it evokes. Its triggers can be life-shaking experiences that require us to reassess and reorganize our thoughts and priorities. The purpose of sadness is to get us to slow down and enter a space of deep reflection.

212

Welcome sadness

Try this when
you need to pause
and reflect

You will need
Paper, watercolours,
paintbrush, pen

15 minutes

Draw a cloudy landscape and paint using different shades of grey, then write down what these clouds could represent for you.

SELF-REFLECTION Does the landscape look like a heavy storm or is it lighter than expected? Could this signify that your sadness is bigger or smaller than you thought? Do you need space to sit with it, or do you feel you need to talk to someone about it?

213

The boulder
we carry

Try this when
you're feeling weighed
down by sadness

You will need
Paper, coloured pencils

15 minutes

Sadness is often accompanied by a sense of heaviness. Draw a person dragging a boulder up a hill. Be as detailed or as simplified as you wish. Take a moment to reflect on what's weighing you down. Inside the boulder, write down the things that feel heavy for you right now using coloured pencils.

SELF-REFLECTION How big is the boulder? Could this be a realistic representation of how you are currently experiencing your burdens? What could help lighten the load?

214

The cave

Try this when
you want to better
understand your feelings

You will need
Paper, coloured pencils

15 minutes

Sadness is a time for reflection and introspection. Draw yourself inside a cave, then surround the page with thought bubbles and write down what you might be thinking while secluded within it.

SELF-REFLECTION How scary was it to draw yourself on your own in a cave? Might you be afraid of being alone with your own thoughts? Are there many things you need space to think about? If this exercise feels overwhelming, you can talk to an art therapist.

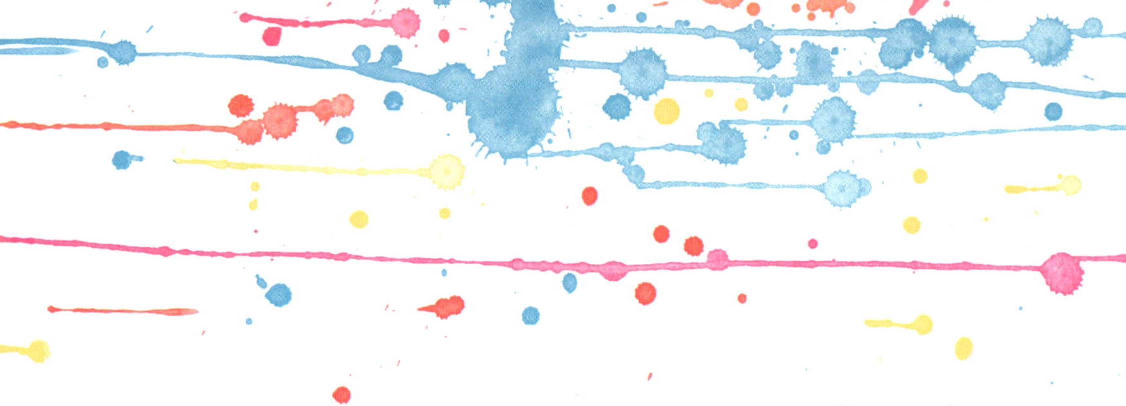

215

Tears can be waterfalls

Try this when
you want to identify
what is making you sad

You will need
Paper, coloured pencils, pen

20 minutes

Draw a face to fill a piece of paper, then draw teardrops falling from the face. Inside each teardrop, write down what you are sad about. When you've finished, take a moment to write what this sadness could be trying to teach you about yourself.

SELF-REFLECTION Did you cry while performing this exercise? We sometimes disconnect our body from our feelings, so we can always benefit from mindfully connecting back to them. Were you able to identify different reasons for your sadness? What lessons did your sadness bring?

216

My sadness guide

Try this when
you want to see sadness
in a new light

You will need
Paper, coloured pencils

15 minutes

Think of an animal, real or imaginary, that represents your sadness, and draw it. Think about this creature's strengths and weaknesses. Reflect on whether this animal is here to accompany you when you are sad, or if it is here to help you overcome sadness.

SELF-REFLECTION Is your chosen animal scary or friendly? Could this reflect your current relationship with sadness? What strengths does the animal possess? Might these provide clues that could help you manage your sadness?

217

Embodying sadness

Try this when
you want to explore where
sadness lives inside you

You will need
Non-toxic watercolours
or lipstick, paintbrush

15 minutes

Embodying a feeling means experiencing it not
just in your mind, but also in your body. If you feel
comfortable, close your eyes and notice where
you hold sadness physically. Once you've located
that spot, gently draw a heart on it using non-toxic
watercolours or lipstick. Take a moment to observe
your experience with curiosity, holding that feeling
with compassion instead of judgement.

SELF-REFLECTION Did drawing on your body help
integrate the emotional experience? How was it to
hold a difficult feeling with love and compassion?
Could you build more space for yourself to explore
this discomfort through creativity?

218

Take a sad song

Try this when
you are ready to face
difficult emotions

You will need
Music device, paper, pencil

10 minutes

Sometimes, the only way through discomfort is to sit
with it, since pushing it away often makes it stronger.
Find a song that makes you feel sad, and while you
listen to it, draw a line that follows the song's rhythm
on some paper.

SELF-REFLECTION How difficult was it to sit with
sadness for the length of the song? Did sitting with
the feeling change how you experienced it? If you
quickly switched songs, could it be that you are
avoiding this feeling as it is too uncomfortable?

219

Me and loneliness

Try this when
you want to understand how
loneliness affects you

You will need
Paper, pencil, coloured pencils

20 minutes

When you strenuously avoid feeling
lonely, you may try to distract yourself
or seek connectivity from a sense of
urgency rather than authenticity, causing
you to feel even more disconnected.
Embracing loneliness can be done
through gentle curiosity. Fold a piece
of paper in half, and on one side of the
page, draw what loneliness feels or
looks like to you. It could be an empty
chair, a solitary figure, or an isolated
object. On the other side, draw yourself
sitting next to that image, offering
comfort or support in whatever way
feels right to you.

SELF-REFLECTION How did it feel to
externalize loneliness? Did it make
you feel more alone, or were you
relieved? Were you able to provide
comfort? Do you ever intentionally
schedule time to be alone?

220

Holding heaviness
in your heart part 1

Try this when
you want to explore your sadness

You will need
Stone, timer, paper, pencil

10 minutes

Go outside and find a stone to represent
your sadness, taking note of things like
its size, texture, colour, and whether it's
cracked or chipped. Set a timer for
3 minutes and explore the stone with
curiosity. Notice the sensation of the
weight in your hands, feel the texture,
and take a deeper look at the colours or
patterns within it. When the timer stops,
take a moment to reflect on the physical
qualities you noticed and use these as
inspiration to write down what this stone
says about your sadness.

SELF-REFLECTION How big was your
stone? Did it feel heavy or light? If it
was light, could it be that your sadness
isn't as bad as you think? Or could this
reflect a tendency to minimize this
feeling? Are there any parallels between
the stone and your sadness? Is it heavy,
multilayered, or dark? Is it light, smooth,
or translucent?

221

Holding heaviness in your heart part 2

Try this when
you're in need of comfort

You will need
Stone, paint, paintbrush

10 minutes

Take the stone from the previous exercise or choose a new one. On one side of the stone, paint a symbol that represents your sadness. On the other side, paint a symbol that represents comfort. While the paint dries, reflect on what needs to happen for your sadness to feel lighter. Keep this stone somewhere where it will remind you that you can hold your feelings and heal them at the same time.

SELF-REFLECTION Was it hard or easy to find comforting things to help you? Do you need to shift how you are performing self-care, or do you need to increase your connectivity with others?

222

The bonfire

Try this when
you're ready to let go of sadness

You will need
Paper, markers, pencil, paint, paintbrush

20 minutes

Gazing into a campfire is a perfect way to reflect and ready yourself to let things go. With a marker, draw logs stacked as though you were going to start a fire. Then, using a light pencil, write down on top of the logs all the things that make you sad and you wish you could let go of. Paint colourful flames above your words and imagine your sadness and worries burning away with the fire.

SELF-REFLECTION How did it feel to see the feelings fade away? Was it liberating or difficult? Could this be a sign that there are certain thoughts you are ready to let go of? Or are there still things you need more time to reflect on, even if they feel uncomfortable?

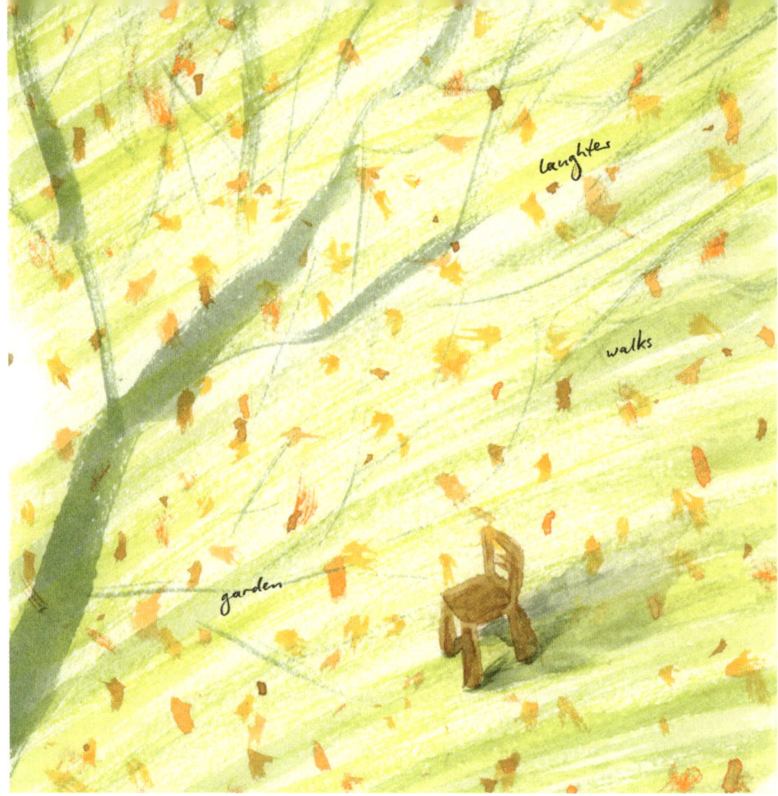

223

The empty
chair drawing

Try this when
you need a gentle way
to remember

You will need
Paper, markers, pencil,
watercolours, paintbrush

20 minutes

When you experience loss, whether through death
or suddenly no longer having something you held
dear, you need space to hold the grief that comes
with it. Paint your favourite chair and leave it empty.
Add symbols or words that represent what you miss
the most about the person, pet, or thing you have
lost around the outside using paint or markers.

SELF-REFLECTION How does it feel to stare at the
empty chair? Was it easy to write down what you
miss, or did you find it difficult? Be gentle with
yourself – no loss is ever easy to bear.

NOTE Depending on the type of loss, the grieving
process can be difficult to navigate. Be mindful that,
while these exercises can help, this is a journey best
approached with an expert.

224

Memory collage

Try this when
you're ready to start
processing your loss

You will need
Paper, photos, magazine or
printed images, markers,
scissors, glue

30 minutes

Processing grief is about learning to love something in a different way. Create a collage that represents memories of the person, pet, or thing you have lost. When you are done, look at your collage and take some time to reflect on what mattered to you most about that connection.

SELF-REFLECTION Was it easy or difficult to sit with past memories? If tears come, allow them to readily flow. Are there things you miss that you might be able to recreate for yourself or someone else?

225

The healing box

Try this when
you need comfort
and support

You will need
Paper, markers, pencil,
paint, paintbrush

20+ minutes

Draw a box and decorate it with symbols that represent love. If you wish, you can use a real box. Inside the box, write notes or paint small symbols that bring you peace, support, or help with honouring your grief. Do this exercise in one sitting, or add to it as ideas come to you.

SELF-REFLECTION What helps comfort you the most? Do you have access to it? Did you add things you have used in the past, or are there new things to integrate? In times of grief, it is especially important to make room for self-care.

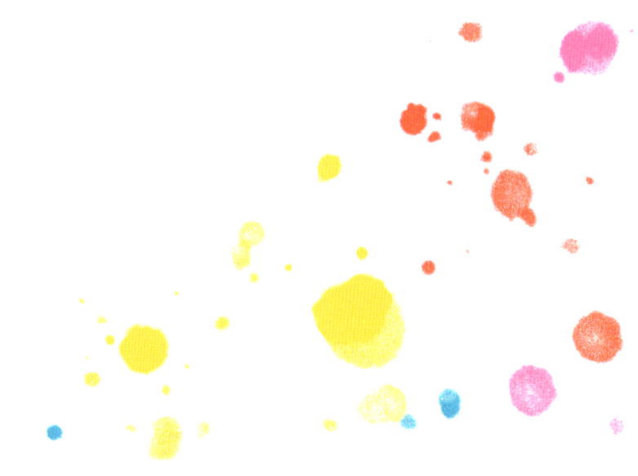

226

From rain
to rainbow

Try this when
you feel like giving up

You will need
Paper, markers, pencil,
watercolours, paintbrush

15 minutes

Good things can come out of adversity if you're
able to observe difficulties with openness and
compassion, and allow yourself to connect with
others. Paint a cloud to represent your sadness.
Then, imagine the weather changing and paint the
sun appearing. Finally, paint a rainbow. Write down
what is making you sad next to the cloud, then write
who or what the sun might represent. To finish, write
all the things you could learn from this exercise next
to the rainbow.

SELF-REFLECTION How did it feel to acknowledge your
sadness? What does the rainbow symbolize for you?
Did you identify anyone who can support you
through difficult times?

227

Joyful reframe

Try this when
you need to find
strength in sadness

You will need
Book, paper, pencil,
markers, coloured pencils

20 minutes

Skim through the pages of a book and try to identify
words that represent sadness for you, then write
them down. Use these words to write a poem or
reflection where you transform them into a message
of joy, hope, or strength. Finally, decorate it with
drawings that reinforce their message.

SELF-REFLECTION Was it difficult to transform sad
words into something positive? What did you notice
that helped you shift the negative into something
encouraging? Was there anything that emerged
unexpectedly that made you feel joyful?

228

What brings me joy?

Try this when
you want to connect
with happiness

You will need
Favourite art materials

20 minutes

Using your favourite materials, draw or paint a heart the size of the page. Inside the heart, draw symbols or write words that represent what and who make you the happiest.

SELF-REFLECTION Was it hard or easy to identify what brings you joy? Do you incorporate these things into your daily life? Or are there things that are just saved for special occasions?

229

There's wisdom in joy

Try this when
you need to lift your spirits

You will need
Paper, watercolours,
paintbrushes, markers

20 minutes

Wet a piece of paper, then fill the page in colours that bring you happiness. While it dries, search through books or online for quotes that bring you happiness. When your painting is dry, write these down over the top.

SELF-REFLECTION Did you already know what quotes you wanted to use, or did you find new ones? Are the colours you chose your usual happy colours? If they are, make sure to integrate them into your everyday life, perhaps through clothing or accessories.

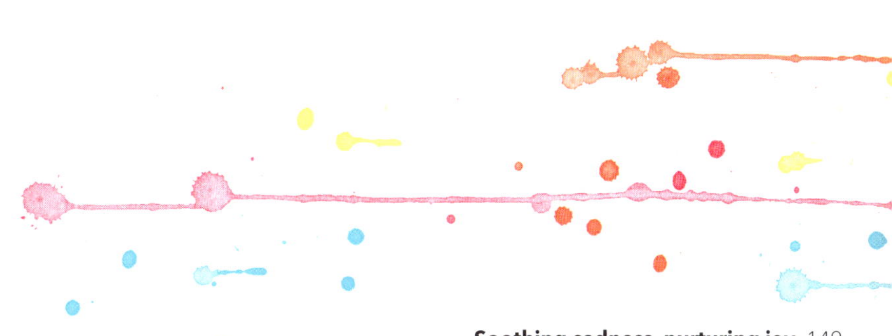

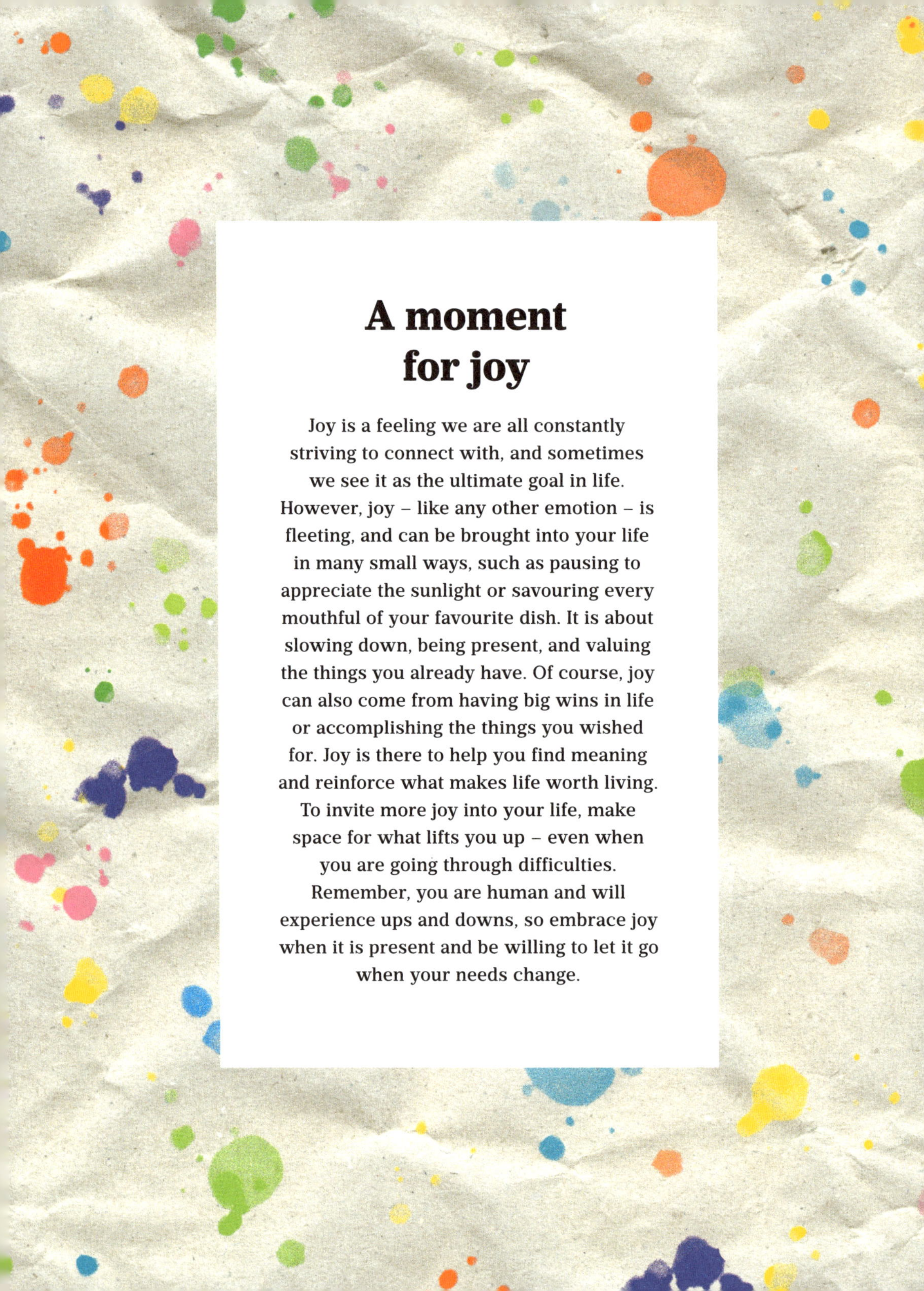

A moment for joy

Joy is a feeling we are all constantly striving to connect with, and sometimes we see it as the ultimate goal in life. However, joy – like any other emotion – is fleeting, and can be brought into your life in many small ways, such as pausing to appreciate the sunlight or savouring every mouthful of your favourite dish. It is about slowing down, being present, and valuing the things you already have. Of course, joy can also come from having big wins in life or accomplishing the things you wished for. Joy is there to help you find meaning and reinforce what makes life worth living. To invite more joy into your life, make space for what lifts you up – even when you are going through difficulties. Remember, you are human and will experience ups and downs, so embrace joy when it is present and be willing to let it go when your needs change.

230
Joyful artists

Try this when
you want to explore how art influences your emotions

You will need
Favourite art materials

30 minutes

Surrounding yourself with art that improves your mood can foster emotional wellbeing. Think about which artists bring you joy and look for examples of their work. Observe what these artists might have in common with you. Is it their preference for certain colours or themes, or their composition? Finally, create an artwork using these common elements.

SELF-REFLECTION Which artists did you find uplifting? Do you already have some of their art hanging in your home? If you don't, could you start adding them now? Were you able to create a sympathetic artwork? How did it make you feel?

231
The joy chain

Try this when
you want to brighten up your day

You will need
Pen, stapler, colourful strips of paper (a thumbs width, and the length around your wrist)

30+ minutes

Think of at least ten good deeds you can do to make others happy and write them on strips of paper. Staple the first one to form a circle, then do the same with the rest, ensuring the strip goes through the circle first so you form a paper chain. See how long you can make your chain.

SELF-REFLECTION Did you choose simple acts, or were they complicated? Could this be a reflection of how you see your own happiness? Did making others happy help improve your mood? What was your favourite thing, and could you do it more often?

Happy place map

Try this when
you want to explore
what makes you happy

You will need
Favourite art materials

20+ minutes

Think about your happy place, then draw a map to represent it. Begin with an outline of the area: is it a room, a building, or somewhere in nature? Then, include the details that make it special for you – perhaps there's a quiet corner, a place for being with family or friends, or an area where you can experience freedom and unconditional love.

SELF-REFLECTION Does just looking at this space already make you smile? Could this happy place be projecting the things you need to include in your daily life? When you are feeling sad or experience other uncomfortable feelings, can you look back to this as a source of comfort and inspiration?

Joyful self-portrait

Try this when
you need a reminder of the
good you bring to others

You will need
Paper, watercolours,
paintbrushes, coloured
pencils, mirror

15+ minutes

Place a mirror in front of you and draw a rough sketch of yourself. Then, imagine yourself sharing positivity with the world. Around your self-portrait, paint images or symbols that show positive vibes radiating into the world around you.

SELF-REFLECTION How does it feel to view yourself as a source of joy for others? Do you see yourself this way, or are you feeling doubtful that this could be you? If you do feel dubious, could you consider talking to an art therapist or other specialist?

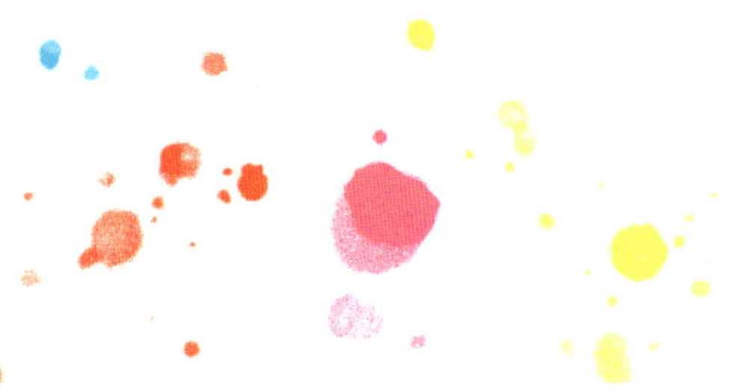

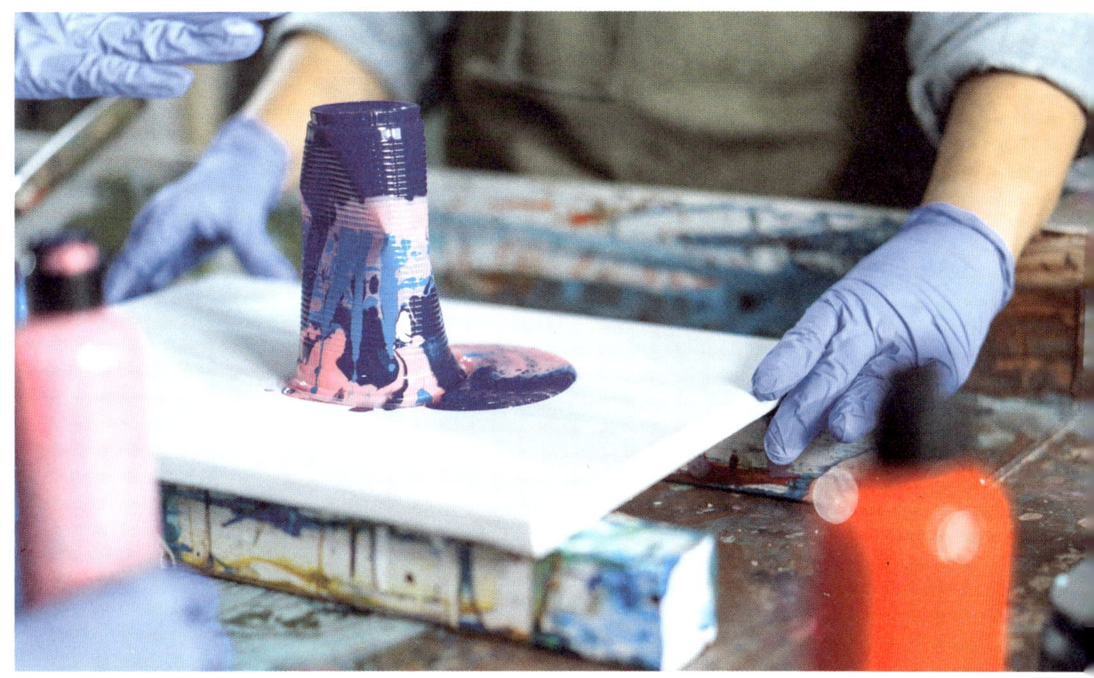

234

Playful art

Try this when
you want to connect
with your inner child

You will need
Paint, cup, cardboard
or small canvas

15+ minutes

If you have anxiety about making a mess, this project may be triggering for you, but approach the process with a playful curiosity. Prepare an area where you can potentially make a mess without worrying. Think of a colour that makes you smile, then pour some of that colour paint into a cup. Cover the top of the cup with a piece of cardboard or canvas, lift the cup up, turn it upside down – keeping the card or canvas in place – and quickly put it back down. Watch the paint leak out over the cardboard. If you can, play around with the paint to direct it to where you want it to go.

SELF-REFLECTION Was it hard or easy to allow yourself to make a mess? Were you able to connect with your inner child and allow yourself to enjoy the process without worrying about the result? How often do you allow yourself to be wild and carefree?

Happy day

Happiness isn't a perpetual state – it comes and goes. We sometimes need help to reconnect with it, particularly when going through a difficult time. Planning a day that focuses on bringing yourself joy is a great way to give yourself a break and connect with the things that make life worth living.

235 The celebration corner

You will need
Found objects, pen, paper

First, find a small personal corner in your home where you can display some found objects – natural materials, such as stones and shells, small tokens, or mementos that remind you of all the things you love in your life. Include items, words, or images that bring you happiness and gratitude every day.

236 Happy dance

You will need
Music device, paper, markers

Joy is a high-energy feeling that invites you to move and celebrate. Now, play some music that makes you happy and recalls fond memories. After grooving to a song or two, sit down and grab a marker with each hand, then take them on a dance across a piece of paper.

237 **Food for fun**

You will need
Favourite food items, plate

To continue the flow of a happy day, prepare your favourite meal. Allow yourself to be playful and serve it in a way that feels arty and original.

238 **Comedy prescription**

You will need
Paper, watercolours, paintbrush, coloured pencils, funny film

Next, watch a film that makes you laugh. Either while watching the film or afterwards, write down, paint, or sketch the funniest moments for your own enjoyment.

239 **Scheduling happiness**

You will need
Sticky notes, pen

Finish your day by drawing a happy symbol, such as a smiley sunflower or heart, on a sticky note. Place the note somewhere visible as a reminder that you have the ability to bring joy into your life more often.

SELF-REFLECTION Are there any joyful aspects of your daily life that you frequently overlook? How can you show more gratitude for these? Did any of the objects reveal something new about what makes your life meaningful? Did the music help lift your spirits? How did it feel to create art with both hands simultaneously? Were they moving in the same rhythm and direction? What was it like to play with your food? Did you find comfort in your meal? Were you able to laugh out loud while watching the film? How often do you create opportunities to bring joy into your life? Can reminders be helpful?

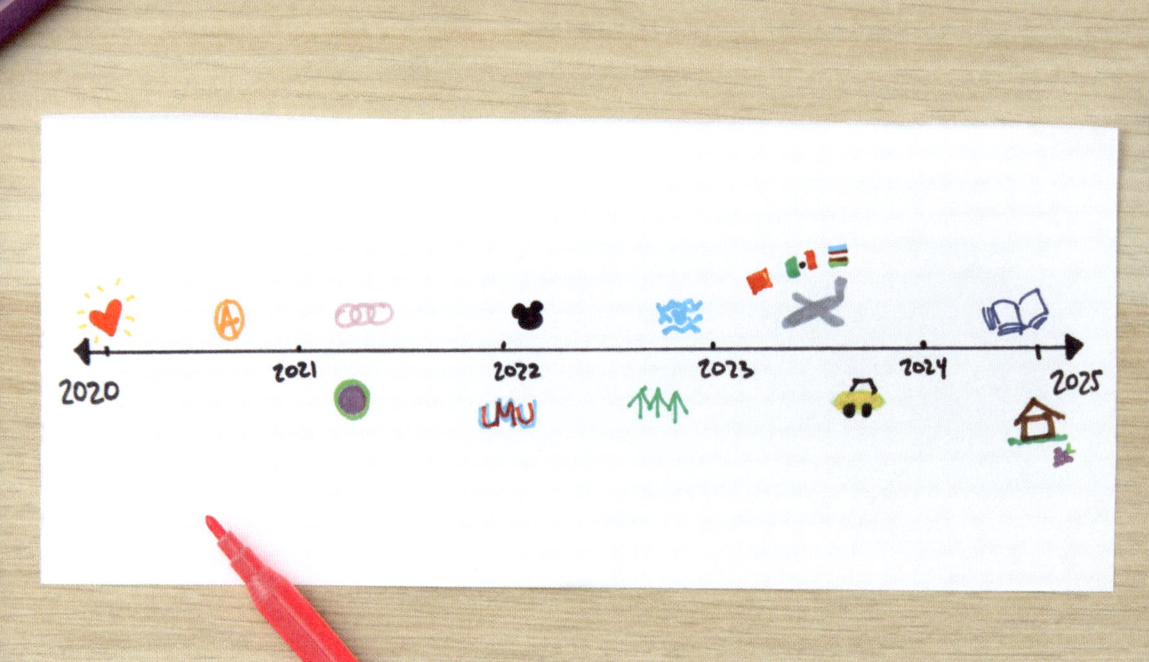

240
Timeline of joy

Try this when
you want to explore what
clouds your happiness

You will need
Paper, markers,
coloured pencils

20 minutes

When you are feeling low, sometimes it can help to
remind yourself of the good times. Draw a line either
horizontally or vertically across a piece of paper to
represent a timeline. Think about the last five years,
then add symbols to the line to represent moments
that brought you the most happiness.

SELF-REFLECTION Have you experienced much joy in
the past five years? If so, celebrate those moments!
If your joyful experiences were few, remember to
honour them, and then reflect on what might have
got in the way of more happiness.

241

Future joy postcard

Try this when
you want to invite more
laughter into your day

You will need
Paper, favourite art materials

15+ minutes

Create a postcard with a funny image
or message for yourself. On the back,
write down a joke or something that
makes you laugh. If you wish, you can
ask a friend or family member to post
this to you when you least expect it, or
you could send it to someone else.

SELF-REFLECTION How would it feel
to receive this postcard in the future?
Do you think it would help lift your
spirits? Do you think it could help
make someone else's day happier?

242

A sculpture full of joy

Try this when
you want to embrace joy

You will need
Found objects, camera

20+ minutes

Look for different objects around your
home that bring you joy, then create
a sculpture with them, honouring your
joyful self. Take a picture of it and allow
this to be a reminder of your inner spark,
letting you know that happiness is all
around you.

SELF-REFLECTION How many objects did
you collect? Did this bring awareness of
how many things are worth celebrating in
your life? Was celebrating your inner joy
easy or difficult?

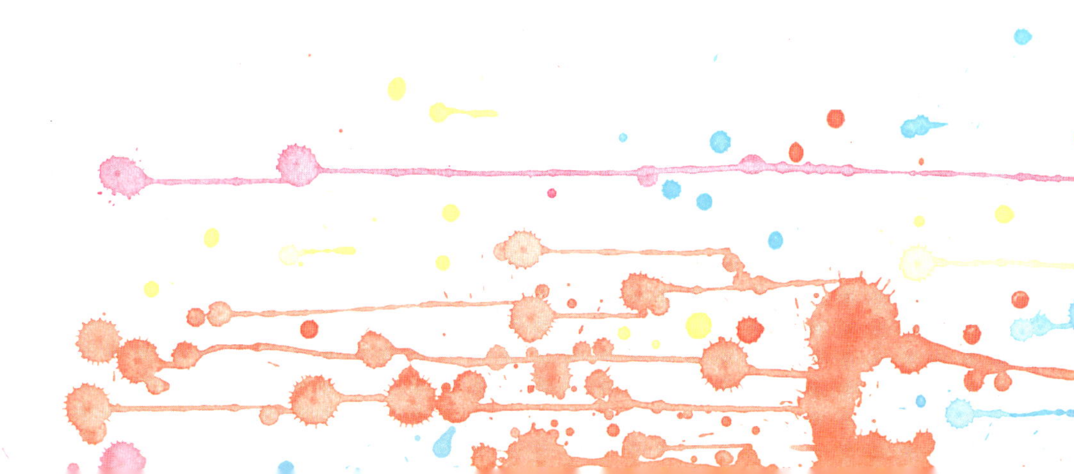

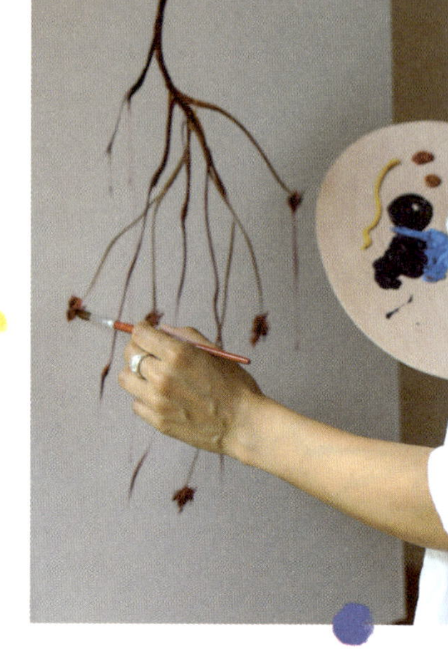

Building emotional resilience

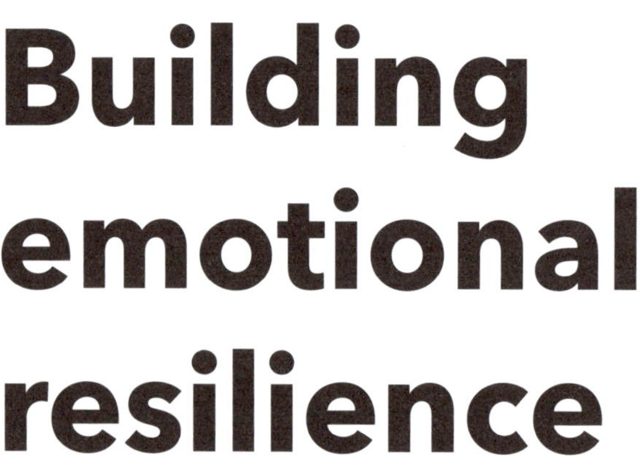

Resilience is one of the most important skills you can develop. It strengthens your ability to take initiative, helps you make wiser decisions, and builds the inner strength needed to face life's inevitable challenges. Resilience doesn't mean that you won't experience difficult emotions – it means you can endure those feelings and bounce back, emerging even stronger than before.

243

I knew, so I did

Try this when
you need confidence
in your own choices

You will need
Paper, pencil, coloured
pencils, markers

15 minutes

Think of a moment where you had a plan to solve
a problem but others advised you against following
it. Draw a symbol to represent the feeling you had
after realizing you were right about following your
intuition and making your own decisions.

SELF-REFLECTION How many moments have you
experienced in your life where following your gut
led to positive outcomes? Was it hard or easy to
make your own choices when there was opposition
to your beliefs? While acting on sound advice is
sensible, remember that trusting your heart can
also lead to positive outcomes.

244

Independence milestones

Try this when
you want to celebrate
your independence

You will need
Paper, watercolours,
paintbrush, pen

20 minutes

Paint a path with stepping stones. Inside each
stepping stone, write down all the things you do
independently, such as cooking, managing your
budget, learning new skills, or keeping active.

SELF-REFLECTION Was it hard or easy to celebrate
small achievements of independence? We can forget
that what seems typical for some of us may not be a
reality for others. Is it possible to use gratitude as a
way to increase your sense of independence?

245

Decision-making part 1

Try this when
you are struggling to make
an important decision

You will need
Paper, pencil, coloured
pencils, markers

20 minutes

Think of a decision you need to make.
Draw six thought bubbles, then assign
one of the following questions to each
bubble and answer each question
according to the decision you are
considering: Does this help me meet
my personal goals or priorities? Will this
build my confidence? Can this help with
my self-care? Does this assist in setting
boundaries? Might this cover a need or a
want? Can this help me become a better
version of myself?

SELF-REFLECTION Do you have a specific
criteria to help you make better decisions?
It might be ensuring your decision aligns
with your core values, or seeking trusted
advice from a loved one. What criteria
do you follow to ensure that you are
making the right choice? Do you listen
to yourself, or do you need the input
of others?

246

Decision-making part 2

Try this when
you feel conflicted between your
intuition and outside opinions

You will need
Paper, pencil, coloured
pencils, markers

15 minutes

Fold a sheet of paper in half. On one side
of the page, draw a head that represents
yourself and add several thought bubbles.
Inside the bubbles, write down your
thoughts about a decision you need
to make. On the other side of the page,
draw more heads with thought bubbles,
and inside these, write down other
people's thoughts about your decisions.
Take a moment to reflect on how these
differ or align with your own thoughts
and why.

SELF-REFLECTION If your thoughts differ
greatly, could it be due to personal
reasons? Sometimes, your unique
life story makes it hard for others to
understand your perspective. How
does it feel when your opinions don't
align with others'? Does it ever shake
your trust in your own intuition?

247

Staying grounded

Try this when
you want to identify what supports your resilience

You will need
Paper, pencil, coloured pencils, markers

20 minutes

Draw a self-portrait where you are standing on the ground, depicting your feet as roots connecting you to the earth. Around the roots, write down what keeps you grounded when you are facing challenging decisions. Maybe it's taking time to meditate, do some journalling, or go for a run.

SELF-REFLECTION Was it difficult to identify activities that keep you emotionally anchored and feeling steady? How often do you engage in these activities?

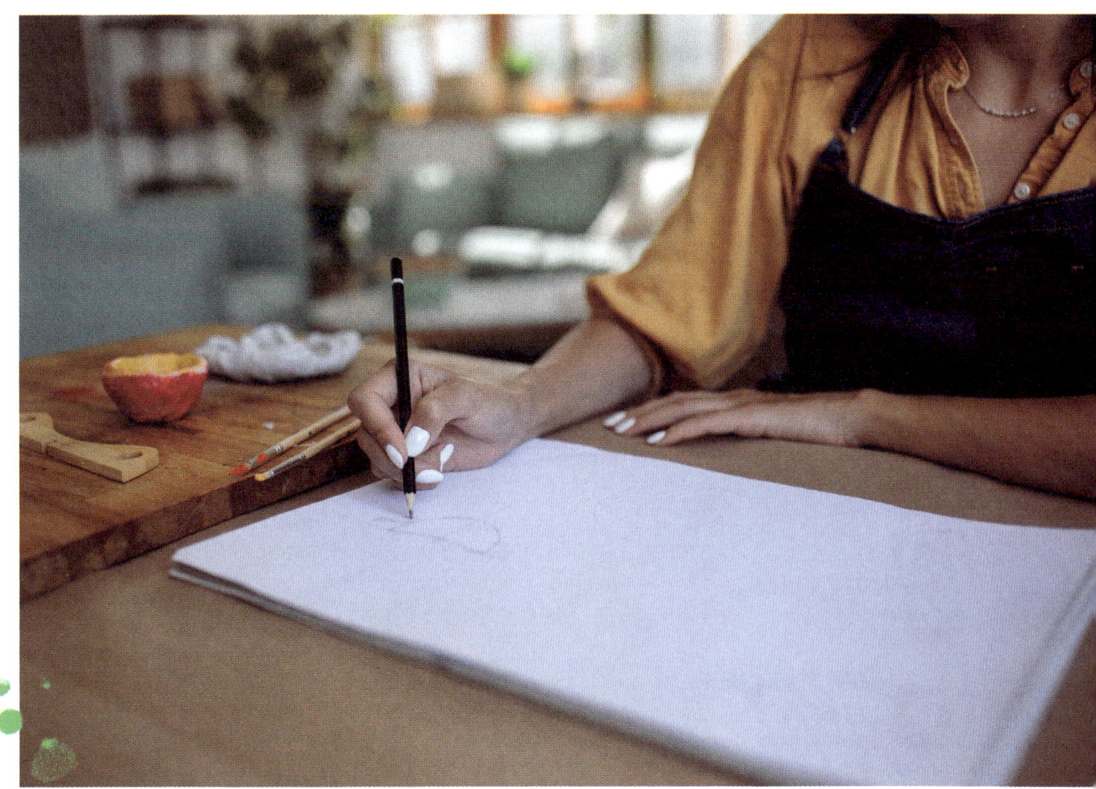

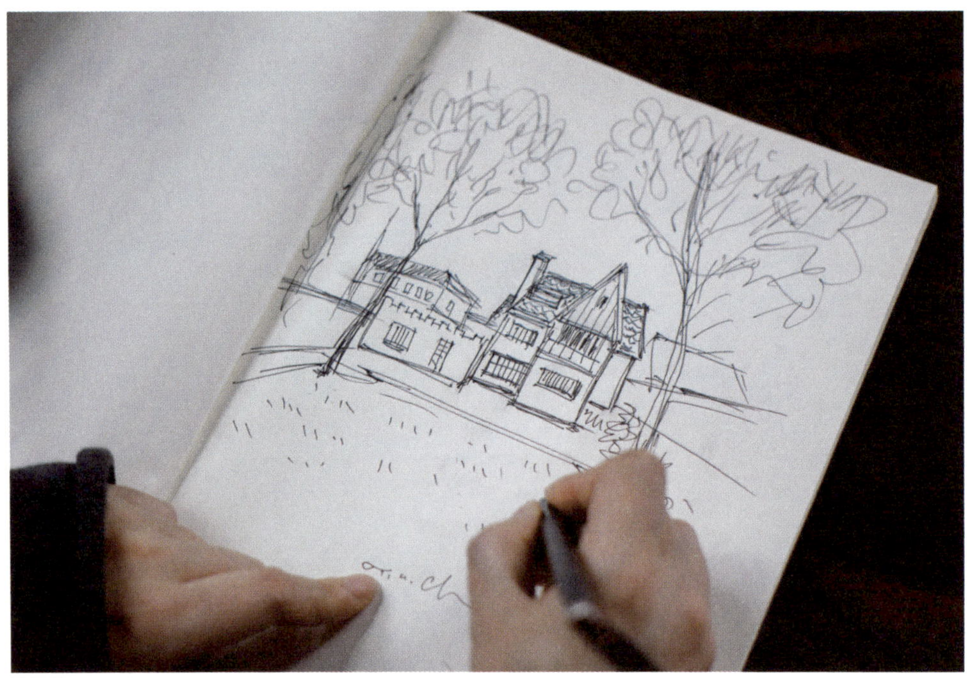

248

Solitude sanctuary

Try this when
you need a break from the
noise of the outside world

You will need
Paper, pencil, coloured
pencils, markers, pen

20 minutes

Draw a peaceful place, imaginary or real, where you
could look forward to spending some time alone.
Add things that might help this space be more
inviting for you, such as a comfy chair, candles,
a favourite mug, or books.

SELF-REFLECTION What does this place offer that
being with others doesn't? Does such a space exist
for you? Or is there a way for you to build a similar
area where you can be on your own and make
independent choices?

249
Alone, not lonely

Try this when
you want to strengthen
your indepedence

You will need
Paper, pencil, coloured
pencils, markers

20 minutes

Independence means learning to be comfortable
with yourself; only then can true resilience be built.
Take time to reflect on a moment where it felt
comfortable to be alone. Perhaps it was when you
were reading your favourite book, or engaged in an
absorbing hobby. Draw this moment to remind
yourself that you can be your best companion.

SELF-REFLECTION Was it hard or easy to identify
moments when you enjoyed being alone? Do you
feel that you need others in order to be content?
Is being with others a way of avoiding being with
your own thoughts?

250
Loneliness
vs solitude

Try this when
being alone feels
uncomfortable

You will need
Paper, pencil, coloured
pencils, markers

20 minutes

Feeling lonely is a difficult emotion to handle and
we can sometimes depend on the company of others
to avoid it. Fold a sheet of paper in half, and on one
side of the page, create a visual representation of
loneliness. It can be abstract or symbolic - an empty
room perhaps, or a bare tree. On the other side of the
page, draw what peaceful solitude could look like.

SELF-REFLECTION Can you picture peaceful solitude,
or is it a concept that is difficult for you to grasp?
Even though connecting with others is crucial, there
should always be space for you as well. How different
were both sides of the paper? Are there things you
can do to promote peaceful solitude and increase
your independence?

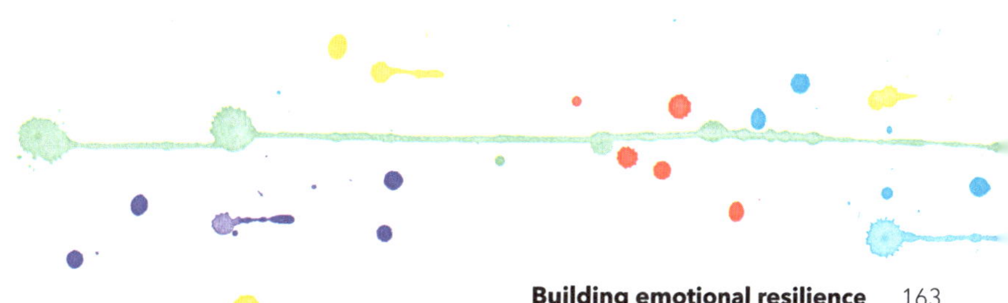

251

Too much independence?

Try this when
you need to practise
asking for support

You will need
Photo of someone
you trust, paper, pen

30 minutes

Trying to handle everything on your own can sometimes leave you feeling isolated. That's why it's important to lean on those you trust. Find a picture of someone you trust and place it in front of you, then write them a letter describing a problem you are having difficulty solving on your own. Once complete, write an imaginary response letter from that person. What would they tell you? Try to use the tone you believe they would use.

SELF-REFLECTION How did it feel to see independence through a different lens? Did sharing your burden help you? Was asking for help difficult? Was it easy to identify someone you could lean on? Remember, you don't have to navigate everything alone, power lies in accepting the need for help.

252

The myth of independence

Try this when
you want to strengthen
your support network

You will need
Paper, pencil,
coloured pencils

25+ minutes

Individuality and self-sufficiency are highly valued, which can lead us to believe we must do everything on our own. However, there is power in collaboration. Reflect on where your ideas about independence come from – it might be family, culture, or the media. Draw two overlapping circles: in one, use symbols to represent your internalized beliefs about self-sufficiency; in the other, depict moments of support or collaboration that brought you strength or relief. In the overlapping section, explore how you might find a balance between these two.

SELF-REFLECTION Where do your beliefs about independence come from? Can you recall moments when collaboration made a positive difference for you? What small steps can you take to invite more support into your life?

A moment for inner strengths

Inner strengths are a vital part of your wellbeing as they not only make your own life better, but they can also help others. They are resources that foster adaptability, vitality, and resilience. When you lean into your strengths, you tend to feel more authentic and energized, and life seems to flow better. Strengths come in many forms and are reflected in the way you think, feel, and behave. While using your strengths to support others is a noble pursuit, it's important to be mindful of overusing them. What happens if you're not available to help at a particular time? Overusing your strengths can lead to burnout, so remember to prioritize your own wellbeing. Taking care of yourself ensures you can continue to give others the support they need.

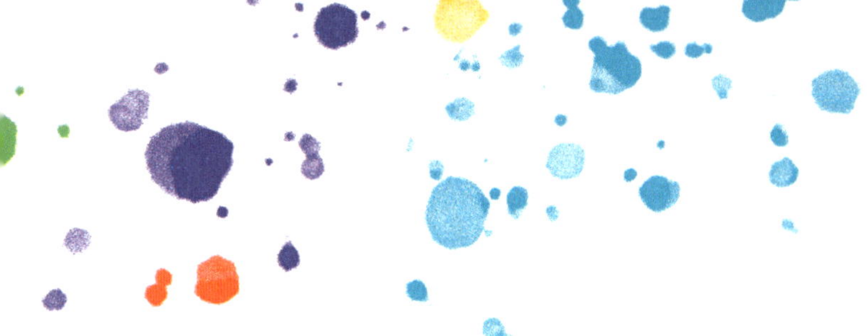

253
What if?

Try this when
fear is holding you back from
starting something new

You will need
Paper, pen, coloured pencils

30 minutes

When considering whether to start
something new, it's normal to feel afraid
because our brains naturally gravitate
towards negative thinking – this is an
evolutionary trait designed to keep
us vigilant to danger. Draw a thought
bubble in the middle of a page, and think
of a project you want to begin. Inside the
bubble, draw all the positive things that
could happen if everything worked out in
your favour.

SELF-REFLECTION Was it easy or hard to
imagine positive outcomes? Did thinking
about things working out become more
worrisome than hopeful, or the opposite?
Sometimes, we can be more afraid of
success than failure. Notice if this is what
could be getting in the way of taking
your first steps towards something.

254
Up for a challenge?

Try this when
you're ready to take
small steps towards change

You will need
Paper, pen, coloured pencils

30+ minutes

Draw seven squares to represent the
days of the week, colouring them in if
you wish. Inside each square, write down
one new thing you want to try for a week
and commit to doing it. It can be a dish
to try out, or a different way to commute
to work. Practising initiative in small ways
can help us take bigger steps. It can also
show us that good things come from
trying something new.

SELF-REFLECTION How did it feel to take
the lead in trying new small things for
yourself? Were you able to complete all
seven challenges? If you still struggled
with allowing yourself to try new things,
what do you think got in the way?

255
The whimsical to-do list

Try this when
you are lacking motivation

You will need
Paper, watercolours,
paintbrush, pencil, stickers

30+ minutes

We sometimes need motivation to start
making changes in our lives. Paint a piece
of paper with colours that feel soothing
and inviting. As it dries, write down five
things you have been meaning to do for
a while. It can be as small as doing the
laundry. Use imagery to represent the
things you want to do and decorate it
in a way that feels fun. Give yourself five
weeks to do what's on this list. When you
complete each task, highlight it using
stickers or by drawing smiley faces.

SELF-REFLECTION Did you have fun
decorating your page? Reframing
things you need to do in a creative
way can make them more enjoyable.
How complicated were the tasks you
gave yourself?

256
The "yes" week

Try this when
you feel like you're in a rut

You will need
Pencil, markers, small notebook

30+ minutes

For one week, keep a small notebook
with you. Each day, notice when an
opportunity, either big or small, presents
itself to you. It could be an invitation, a
new idea, or a chance to try something
different. Choose to say yes to at least
three of them. Make a visual record of the
experience, using symbols or doodles to
represent how it felt to say yes.

SELF-REFLECTION How did it feel to act on
opportunities on the spot? What benefits
were there in taking initiative and being
spontaneous? Could you do this with
bigger opportunities, or is there
something missing?

257

If I dare...

Try this when
you want to build your
self-confidence

You will need
Magazine or image
printouts, paper, glue,
scissors

30 minutes

Make a collage about how your life would look like if
you dared to take the initiative to change something
and put your hesitations aside, such as starting a
dancing class you always dreamed about.

SELF-REFLECTION Does this collage seem attainable,
or does it feel unrealistic? Could your expectations
be getting in the way of taking steps towards
change? Is there any part of the collage that you
already see in your life? Do you hesitate less now
that you can see the possibilities?

258

Your inner fire

Try this when
you're ready to turn
intention into action

You will need
Paper, watercolours,
paintbrushes

20 minutes

Think of a project you have been wanting to start but
haven't yet and write it down, then reflect on what
could help fuel your desire to begin. As you think
of your reasons and motivations, paint a fire and let
it take form intuitively. You can do this painting with
your hands or brushes.

SELF-REFLECTION What's been holding you back from
starting this project? What does this fire represent to
you? What's one small action you can take today to
keep your fire burning brightly?

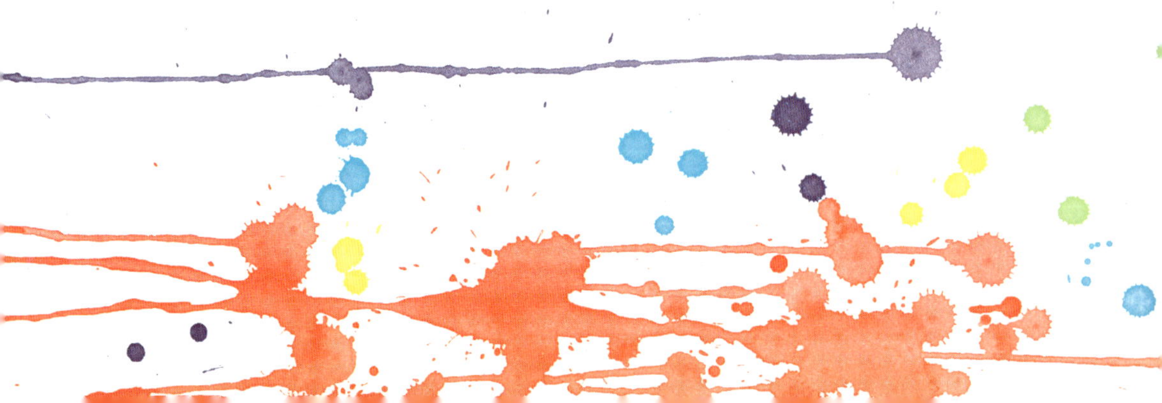

259

Too much initiative?

Try this when
you want to make
better decisions

You will need
Paper, pencil, coloured
pencils, markers

30 minutes

Acting on impulse without proper consideration can sometimes lead to unintended consequences or perceptions of impulsiveness. Divide a sheet of paper into three sections. In the middle section, draw a moment when you used your initiative too quickly. In another section, draw what triggered that action, and in the final section, draw what happened as a result. On the back of the page, reflect on what you could have done differently.

SELF-REFLECTION Would taking a pause before acting have made a difference in that moment? What could help you differentiate between impulsive acts and intentional initiative?

260

Internal traffic light

Try this when
you feel impulsive

You will need
Paper, watercolours,
paintbrushes, markers

20 minutes

Paint a traffic light, then look at the details of your creation. Are the colours uneven? Are there any crooked lines? Note them in your mind's eye. Whenever you realize you want to act too quickly, think of the red light to stop your impulsive behaviour. Think of the yellow light to remind yourself to allow space for reflection, preventing you from making snap decisions; you can always check in with other people to ask for advice. Think of the green light when you are ready to take intentional initiative.

SELF-REFLECTION What situations in your life tend to live in the red light zone? What can you do to make more intentional decisions and avoid impulsive action? Remember to practise the calming exercises in this book to ground yourself before you react.

Daring stories

There are many people around us doing amazing work to make the world a better place, be it celebrities or people you know. Noticing what others are able to accomplish can serve as inspiration for you to go after what you aspire to do.

Try this when
you feel inspired to take action

1 hour 30 minutes

261 **You inspire everyone**

You will need
Paper, pencil, coloured pencils, markers, watercolours, paintbrushes

Think of a famous person you admire who undertakes projects or initiatives to try to positively change the world, then research their life story. How did they start their work? Paint a portrait of this person or some abstract art about their work. Include phrases or quotes, representing what you learned and the inspiration you got from them.

262 **You inspire me**

You will need

Paper, pencil, coloured
pencils, markers,
watercolours, paintbrushes

Next, think about people who are closer to you. Is there a family member, friend, or co-worker that you admire for their positive initiatives? Interview them about what helped them take that first step towards success or change. Find out about their wins and struggles. Then paint a picture of what you admire most about them, adding phrases from their stories.

263 **I am inspired**

You will need

Paper, printed photo
of yourself, markers

Last, write down what you admire about the people who inspire you most. What qualities do they possess? Take a moment to reflect. Then, place a photo of yourself in front of you, and on it write the qualities that you think you could have in common with them. Could you use these attributes to help you kick-start your own projects?

SELF-REFLECTION Are these people's lives markedly similar or different from yours? Could you identify the struggles they faced when using their initiative? From the lessons you learnt here, what can you implement in your own life? Was it easier to relate to someone's experience if they are closer to you? Could you ask them for advice when trying to start a new venture?

264

Don't take yourself so seriously

Try this when
you need to lighten
a heavy mood

You will need
Pencil, markers, printed
photo of yourself, stick–on
googly eyes (optional)

20 minutes

Laughter reduces stress, boosts your mood, and helps build resilience. Appropriately laughing at yourself can even assist in managing pain by giving you a sense of power over your predicament. Place a photo of yourself in front of you, then decorate it to make it look funny. Perhaps paint a silly outfit, give yourself a crazy hat, or add stick-on googly eyes.

SELF-EXPLORATION Does laughing at yourself come easy to you? Or are you afraid of ridicule? Were you able to make yourself laugh with your creation? How does humour help you bounce back from difficult moments?

265

Memes to the rescue

Try this when
life feels overwhelming

You will need
Funny memes, phone
or computer

20 minutes

Laughter is a powerful tool that helps us overcome adversity and navigate life's toughest moments. Think of a challenging situation – whether it's a world event or a personal struggle – and search online for related memes that make you laugh. Either print them out and place them somewhere or make them your screensaver, as a reminder that even in difficult moments there is relief to be found in humour.

SELF-EXPLORATION How does humour help change how you feel about a situation? Does your type of humour reveal how you usually cope with difficulties? Could you use humour as a tool for resilience, not just relief?

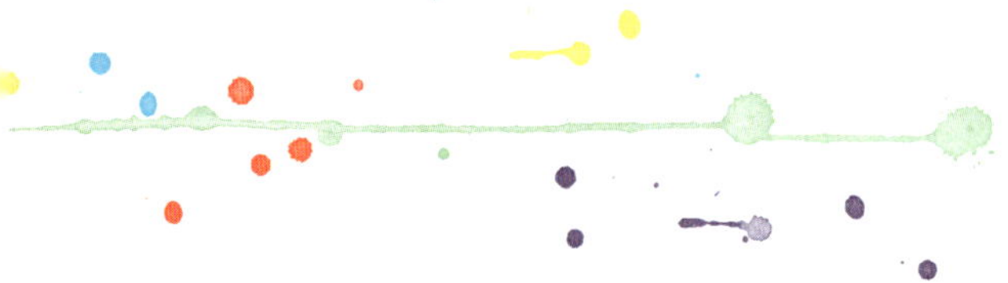

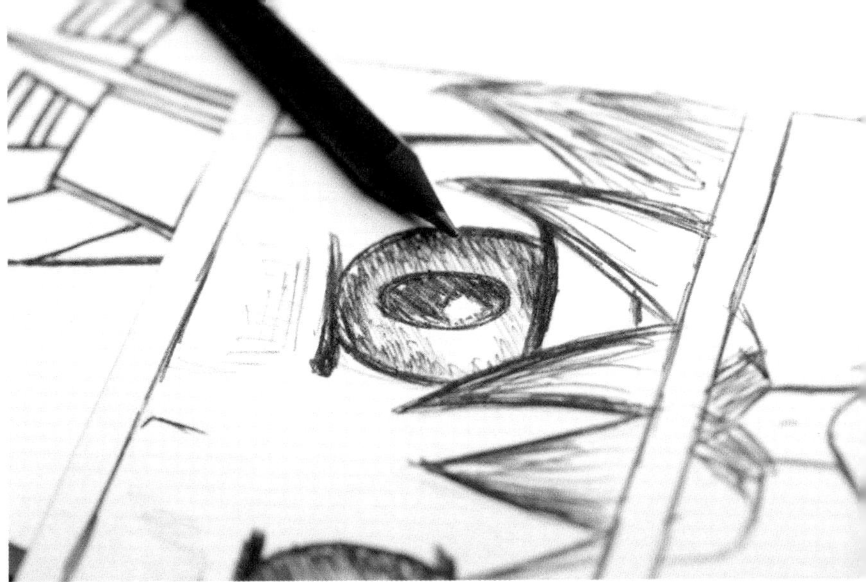

266
Motivational posters

Try this when
you need light-hearted
encouragement

You will need
Paper, watercolours, paintbrushes,
markers, phone or computer

20 minutes

Look for witty motivational quotes and
turn them into posters to hang around
your house so they can cheer you up
during difficult times. Paint them in
decorative letters using joyful colours,
or surround them with funny doodles.

SELF-EXPLORATION Does comical
encouragement help you, or do you
prefer serious advice? Does humour
make you feel better in life?

267
The comic strip

Try this when
you are tired of taking
yourself too seriously

You will need
Paper, markers, coloured pencils

20 minutes

Think of an awkward situation that has
happened to you and draw a humorous
comic strip in three or four scenes.
You can exaggerate moments in order
to tell the story.

SELF-EXPLORATION Was the situation you
found yourself in funny at the time, or
did it become so with hindsight? How
did retelling your story through humour
reframe the experience for you?

268

Ridiculous invention

Try this when
you want to solve your
problems from a new angle

You will need
Paper, pencil, coloured
pencils, markers

15 minutes

Think of an everyday annoyance you experience:
perhaps your coffee always gets cold before you
drink it, or you have seemingly never-ending laundry.
Invent and draw two or three outlandish machines
to solve these problems, such as a robot that follows
you around while keeping your coffee warm. Make
them as crazy and silly as you can.

SELF-EXPLORATION What problem were you trying
to solve in a playful way? Did laughter or absurdity
bring you any relief or insight? Can you use this same
technique to solve bigger problems?

269

Art humour

Try this when
you want to explore
your sense of humour

You will need
Paper, pen

20 minutes

To develop your own sense of humour, explore what
kind of humour you gravitate towards. Look around
for some amusing art, and try to notice what things
you like or find most amusing. Is it when something is
grossly exaggerated? When things are unexpected?
Is it especially sarcastic? Make a note of them.

SELF-EXPLORATION Do you think the type of humour
you like is appropriate? Or do you feel it's too dark?
Could this be preventing you from taking advantage
of humour to cope with your difficulties?

270

Join the laughter

Try this when
you want to replace sadness
with laughter

You will need
Paper, coloured pencils,
markers, phone or computer

20 minutes

Did you know that it is easier for us to laugh in groups than to laugh alone? Laughing is contagious! Organize a comedy evening with friends or family, and watch a funny film or a stand-up comedy show. Before people arrive, draw how you are feeling at that moment. After they leave, draw another picture showing how you are feeling, then compare both drawings.

SELF-EXPLORATION Did your artwork change after spending time laughing with others? Was the act of laughing enough to help improve your mood? Or did laughing with others help to amplify the humorous moment?

271

Add humour to your to-do list!

Try this when
you want to improve your
daily mood

You will need
Paper, coloured pencils,
markers, pen, small
notebook

20 minutes

To develop your sense of humour, you need to stimulate it. Try to do something that makes you laugh daily for a week. Perhaps watch a funny TV show or learn a new joke. Each time, write down what made you laugh, then draw an emoji next to it to capture your mood. On the final day, look at how your mood progressed over the week.

SELF-EXPLORATION Did you learn something new about your sense of humour? Did it feel harder to laugh some days than others? Why? How can integrating humour into your life help you cope through difficult times?

Too much humour? Part 1

Try this when
you use laughter to mask difficult emotions

You will need
Paper, coloured pencils, markers, pen, small notebook

20 minutes

Even though a sense of humour is a great strength, if used inappropriately it can backfire. Overusing it might lead people to think you are deflective and unable to deal with difficult subjects or emotions. To help keep it in check, draw a mask that's laughing, then decorate it with symbols that represent how humour can shield your emotions, such as an umbrella to protect you from emotional storms. Inside, write or draw symbols representing the feelings that humour could be trying to mask.

SELF-EXPLORATION How does humour protect you? Do you use it appropriately, or is it becoming a shield or mask you hide behind? What feelings does humour conceal? Could you benefit from working with those feelings? Remember, you can reach out to an art therapist if these feelings become overwhelming.

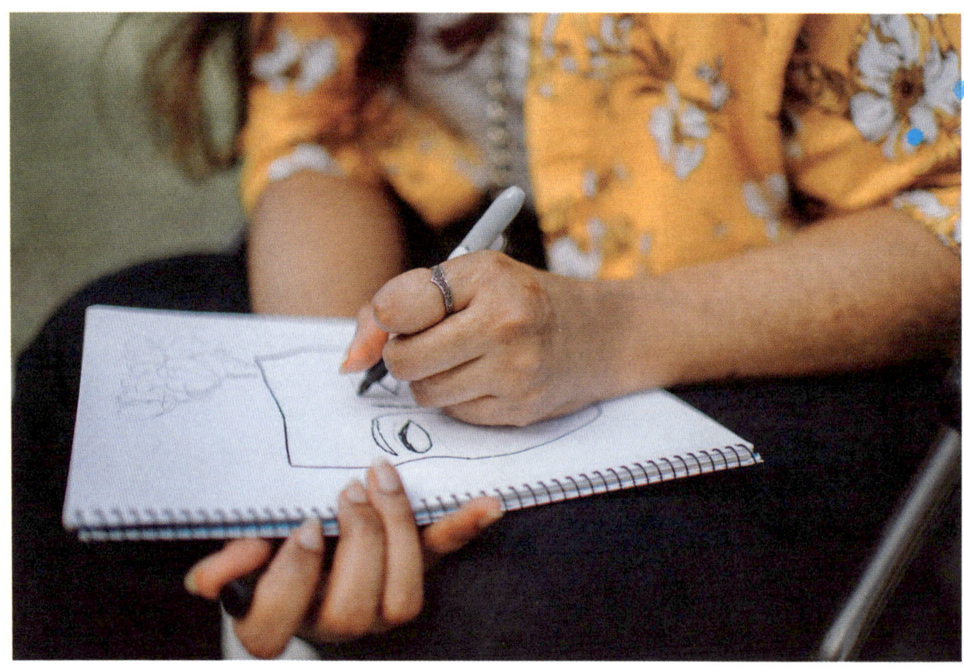

273

Too much humour? Part 2

Try this when
you use humour inappropriately

You will need
Paper, coloured pencils,
markers, pen

20 minutes

Draw a mask that looks sad. Think of
a time when your use of humour might
have led to misunderstandings or hurt.
Then behind the mask, write down what
feelings humour could have been hiding
for you.

SELF-EXPLORATION What feelings were
you trying to avoid when using humour
inappropriately? Do you find these
feelings difficult? Could working through
the exercises in this book help you with
your emotional expression instead of
relying on humour to manage them?

274

We've all been there

Try this when
you want to find humour in
shared struggles

You will need
Magazine or image printouts,
paper, markers, scissors, glue,

20 minutes

Look for images that represent everyday
problems we all have, such as being in a
traffic jam or spilling milk, then glue them
on to some paper. Add captions to the
pictures that make fun of the situation,
and share them with others if possible.
For example, you could add "Taking the
need to slow down very seriously over
here" to the image showing being stuck
in stationary traffic.

SELF-EXPLORATION How does finding
funny phrases for shared experiences
help you reframe life's challenges?
Is using humour a good tool to connect
with others for you? Did humour help
you feel less alone?

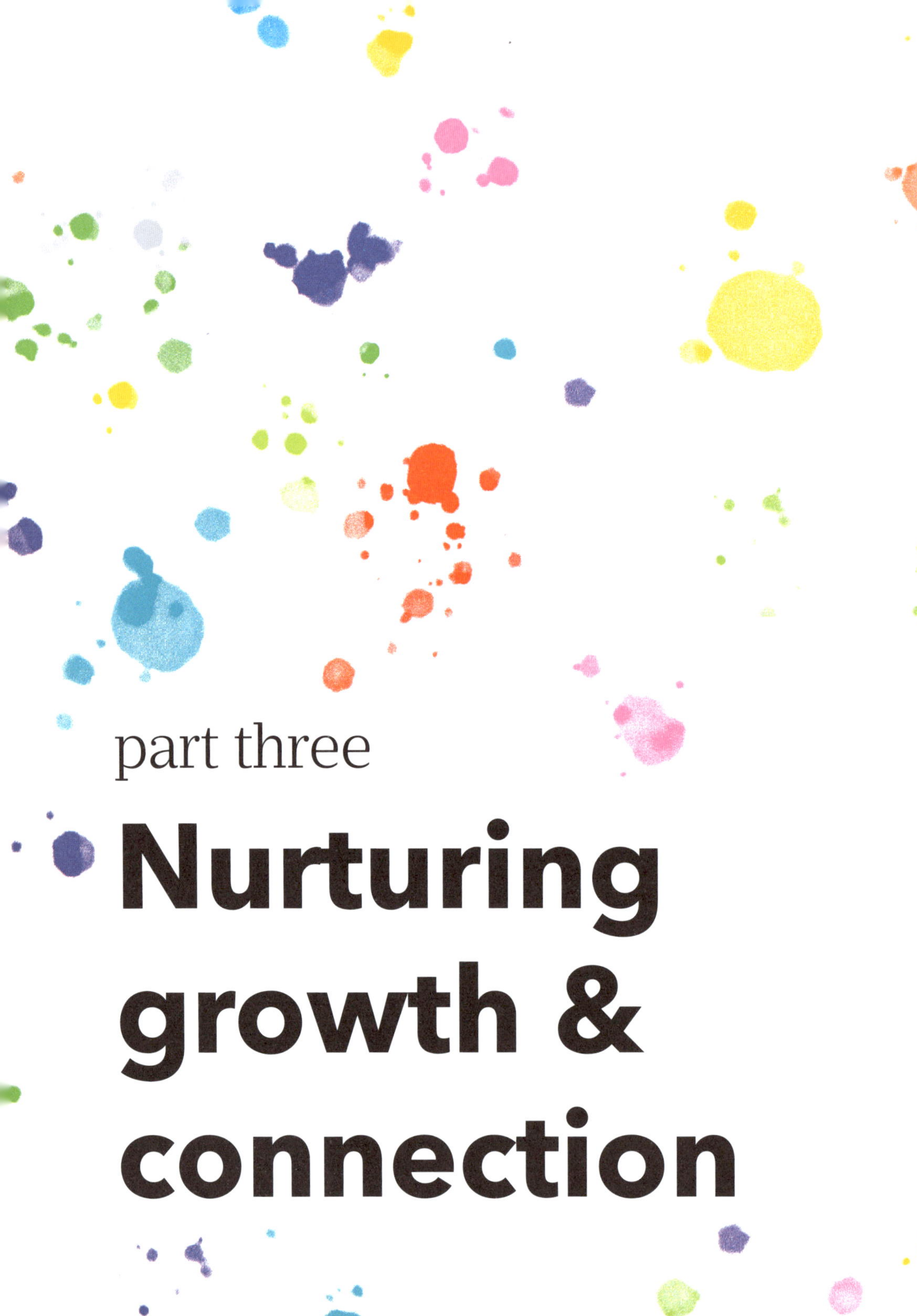

part three
Nurturing growth & connection

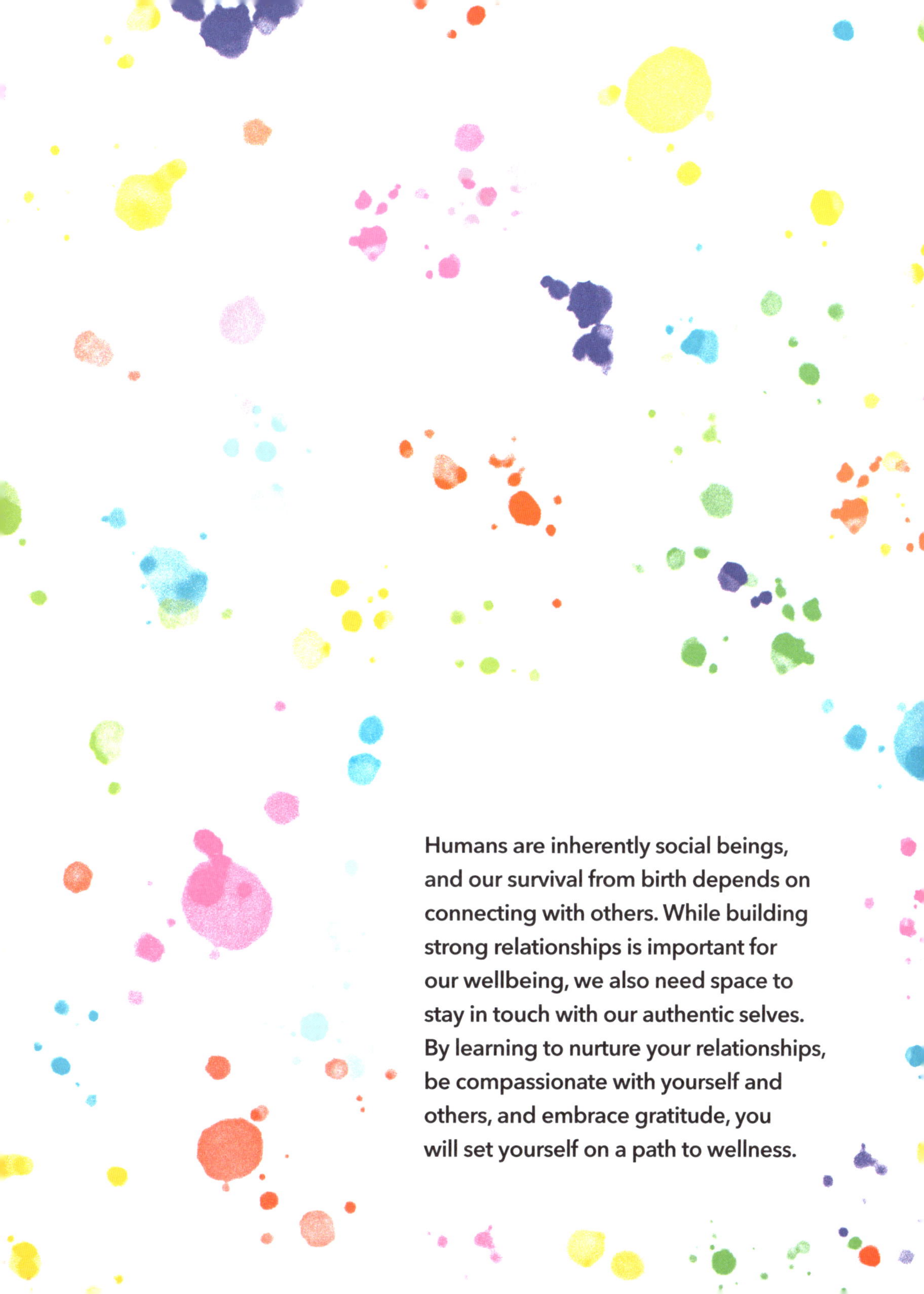

Humans are inherently social beings, and our survival from birth depends on connecting with others. While building strong relationships is important for our wellbeing, we also need space to stay in touch with our authentic selves. By learning to nurture your relationships, be compassionate with yourself and others, and embrace gratitude, you will set yourself on a path to wellness.

Healing & growing relationships

Relationships deeply impact our emotions and have the power to either uplift us or increase our burdens. In this chapter we will explore how art can help us navigate the complex world of human connections. You will discover how to identify support systems, foster positive connectivity, and establish healthy boundaries to protect your personal wellbeing.

275

Social landscape

Try this when
you want to reflect on your
key relationships

You will need
Paper, pencil, coloured
pencils, markers,
watercolours, paintbrushes

20+ minutes

Create a garden scene using the following ideas as inspiration. Allow the earth to represent people who have influenced your values and morals. Create trees to symbolize social connections that serve as pillars in your life. Paint or draw flowers to represent those who make your life beautiful. Add gardening tools to indicate people that help build you up and make you a better person.

SELF-REFLECTION Were any names repeated throughout the different parts of your creation? Could they be the most important people in your life? How diverse are your groups? How many were family, friends, and school or work relationships?

276

You + me = US

Try this when
you want to explore the
depth of a close relationship

You will need
Paper, pencil, watercolours,
paintbrushes, pen

30+ minutes

Think of someone you love deeply. Draw a circle to represent yourself and another circle that overlaps it to represent this person. You can colour them with your favourite colours. Inside your circle, write down what you give to the other person, and in their circle, write down what they give to you. Where the circles intersect, write down any goals and interests that you both share.

SELF-REFLECTION Was there a balance between what you both give in this relationship? Or does it seem one person is more invested than the other? What keeps you both connected?

277

Positive relationships
part 1

Try this when
you want to better understand
your relationship expectations

You will need
Paper, magazines and image
printouts, scissors, glue

20+ minutes

When we are in any kind of relationship,
it is important to understand what we
expect from it so that we can check if
our needs are being met. It's also crucial
to know if we might be expecting too
much and sabotaging our relationships.
Create a collage depicting what a
positive relationship looks like for you.
Include images or symbols that represent
not only how they make you feel, but also
how they treat you.

SELF-REFLECTION What did you highlight
as being part of a positive relationship?
Can you find any of those things in
your current relationships? Did your
art include things like respect, support,
and open communication?

278

Positive relationships
part 2

Try this when
you want to explore the quality
of your relationships

You will need
Paper, magazines and image
printouts, scissors, glue

20+ minutes

Create a collage about a current
relationship with someone who is close
to you. Include symbols or images to
represent how you treat them and how
they treat you.

SELF-REFLECTION Is there a big difference
between the previous collage and this
one? How do you treat others when
going through difficulties? How did it
feel to critically explore the quality of
your relationship? If you wish to change
some of the patterns you saw in your
artwork, don't forget that you can reach
out to an art therapist or other specialist.

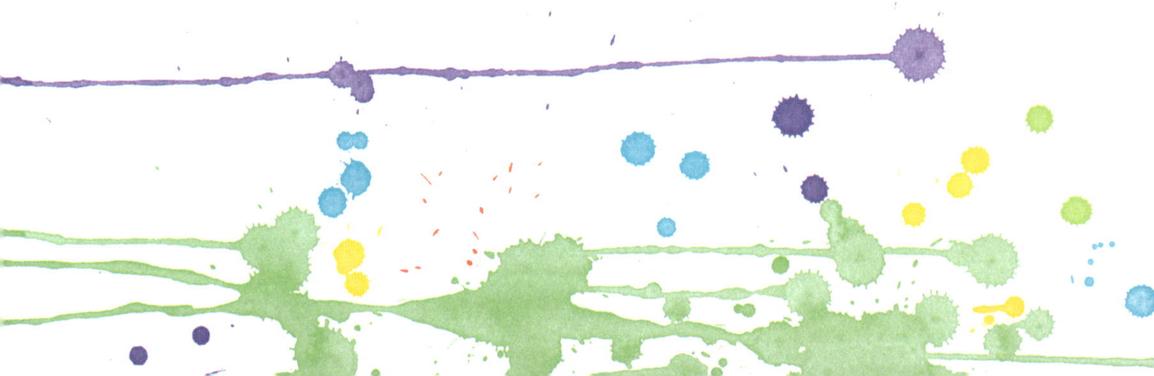

279

Family tree

Try this when
you want to explore
multigenerational patterns

You will need
Paper, pencil, coloured
pencils, markers,
watercolours, paintbrushes

30+ minutes

Sometimes, we might be unconsciously repeating patterns of behaviour that we have inherited from our families. It's important to be aware of and explore these. Draw a family tree, including as many generations as you can. Add three to five things that characterize each family member: maybe a specific profession? A divorce when it wasn't culturally appropriate? If you have living family members who can tell you stories from the past, try to interview them and fill in any gaps.

SELF-REFLECTION Could you find any patterns within your family dynamic? Is there a relative whose life seemed similar to yours? Are there any repetitive behaviours in your family you wish you could change? Could you become the cycle breaker?

280

Shields and vulnerability

Try this when
you want to protect
your heart from others

You will need
Paper plate, watercolours,
paintbrushes

20 minutes

We need to create self-awareness about our fears when entering new relationships. Imagine a paper plate is a shield. On the inside of the plate, use colours or symbols to depict worries, concerns, or triggers you experience when entering new relationships. This might be broken hearts or a black square to represent the unknown. Then on the outside, decorate it with designs that represent what makes you feel safe and able to communicate. Perhaps this is sunlight or simply a soothing colour that represents warmth.

SELF-REFLECTION How did it feel to put your needs first when thinking of relationships? Were you able to identify what helps you feel safe? Are your fears coming from being hurt in a previous relationship? If this is the case, have you considered talking with a trusted friend or a specialist?

281

Misunderstanding timeline

Try this when
you are struggling to resolve conflict in your relationship

You will need
Paper, pencils, markers

30+ minutes

When we get into an argument, it's easy to lose sight of our rational thinking and empathy. However, it is important to learn from mistakes so we can prevent them happening again. Once you have both calmed down, reconnect and create an artwork together. Each draw a timeline in the middle of a page, and use it to reflect on how the conflict started, how it developed, and how it ended. Include words or symbols to represent the story, and take turns to share your timeline without interrupting. Afterwards, note similarities and differences, and focus on understanding each other's perspective. Apologize for mistakes, and identify any lessons learned.

SELF-REFLECTION How did it feel to communicate visually with each other? Did it help bring clarity to the misunderstanding? Were you able to find lessons you could learn from the experience?

282

Build a bridge together part 1

Try this when
you need to better understand your boundaries

You will need
Paper, markers

30+ minutes

Together with the person you are trying to find middle ground with, draw a bridge and each select an end to work on. At your chosen end, write or draw symbols representing your views on the matter. Consider which aspects of your position you are prepared to modify to take the other person's points on board, and note where you prefer not to negotiate. When you are finished, share your perspectives without interruptions. Show gratitude where either party is willing to compromise.

SELF-REFLECTION How did it feel to let go of your own ideas? Was it hard? Sometimes we need to look beyond winning and be flexible in order to make space for relationships to work.

283

Build a bridge together part 2

Try this when
you are ready to
compromise

You will need
Paper, markers

30+ minutes

Now take time to create the centre of the bridge together. Look at each other's non-negotiables, and answer the question, "For you, I am willing to…" Offer ways in which you can help contribute or give space to each other's opinions by drawing or writing about it in the middle.

SELF-REFLECTION How did it feel to put your relationship before your own needs? How does compromising feel for you? Were you speaking honestly, or did you find yourself acting a bit condescending? How did it feel to see the other person offer ways to honour your boundaries?

REMEMBER Being in a positive relationship requires sacrifices to be made from both sides.

284

Portrait of a relationship

Try this when
you are having doubts
about your relationship

You will need
Paper, markers, paper,
computer or phone

20+ minutes

There are times when we may doubt if we should continue certain relationships. Look online for art that represents a conflicting relationship. Once you find a piece, observe it and decide whether the relationship looks like it can be fixed. What would it take to fix it? Is this something you would be willing to do? How about the other person? Focus on being curious and don't try to reach a definitive answer. Decisions are better made when informed and considered, as uncomfortable as it can be.

SELF-REFLECTION Was it uncomfortable to look at your relationship through this lens? Did parts of the image give clarity on how you feel about your relationship? Would it be beneficial to discuss doubts with the person? Relationships are two-sided, so it is crucial to communicate openly before making drastic choices.

285

Two paths

Try this when
you feel conflicted about continuing a relationship

You will need
Paper, uncomfortable art materials, pencil, eraser

30 minutes

Draw two divergent paths, designing the landscape and scenery in any way that feels meaningful to you. On one path, write the pros of staying in the relationship; on the other, write the cons. Once you have finished, stand up and shake off any stress. Then take a moment to reflect on which path aligns more with your needs and values.

SELF-REFLECTION What do the paths look like? Is one more chaotic or more peaceful? Which path feels more *you*? Is your list of pros or cons longer? What do you notice in your body as you look at each path?

286

My future face

Try this when
you're at a crossroads in a relationship

You will need
Paper, pencil, coloured pencils

30+ minutes

Divide a piece of paper in half. On one side, draw a portrait of how you imagine you'll look one year from now if you stay in the relationship. On the other side, draw a portrait of yourself one year from now if you end it. When you have finished, observe both portraits. What do you notice?

SELF-REFLECTION What are the differences? Are they obvious or subtle? Which side looks more at peace, and why do you think that is?

287

Behind the closed door

Try this when
you're seeking closure after a relationship ends

You will need
Paper, pencil, coloured pencils

20+ minutes

Ending a relationship can be heartbreaking – even if it's a bad one. Fold your paper in half, as if creating a greeting card, and keep it closed. On the front, draw a door, and inside, draw five good things that this relationship gave you. It could be great memories or times of support. If possible, imagine sending them love.

SELF-REFLECTION Were you able to hold space for the good things you had in the relationship? Was it painful to think about the positives? Sometimes, connecting to the good can trigger feelings of sadness. Allow your feelings to flow.

288

Letter to your future self part 1

Try this when

you want to imagine the long-term impact of staying in a relationship

You will need

Paper, pen

20+ minutes

Look at the portraits from the future face exercise (page 186). Imagine you chose to stay in the relationship, and write a letter to the version of yourself in that first portrait. In your letter, reflect on what you hope you learnt by staying. What changed within you? What changed in the relationship? What, if anything, stayed the same?

SELF-REFLECTION Does your letter have a positive or negative tone? Could this help give you a sense of how you would feel if you stayed in the relationship? Are there things you could potentially do differently in the relationship?

289

Letter to your future self part 2

Try this when

you want to imagine the long-term impact of ending a relationship

You will need

Paper, pen

20+ minutes

Now, imagine you chose to end the relationship. Write a letter to the version of yourself in the second portrait, reflecting on what you think leaving the relationship would have taught you. What has changed within you?

SELF-REFLECTION Did you feel relief while writing this letter? Could this be a sign it's time to end things? Or did you feel confused? Do you need more clarity from the other person to understand how to move forward?

290

Sunset

Try this when
you want to make peace
with a relationship ending

You will need
Paper, watercolours,
paintbrushes, pen

20+ minutes

Endings can bring beauty into your life. Paint a
sunset on a piece of paper. On the back, write a
letter to the person you ended the relationship with,
highlighting the lessons you learnt throughout your
journey with them. If any unresolved grievances
come up, that's okay, just make sure you end the
letter on a positive note.

SELF-REFLECTION What lessons do you cherish the
most? Are they related to making you a better
person? Does ending this relationship bring
other kinds of opportunities?

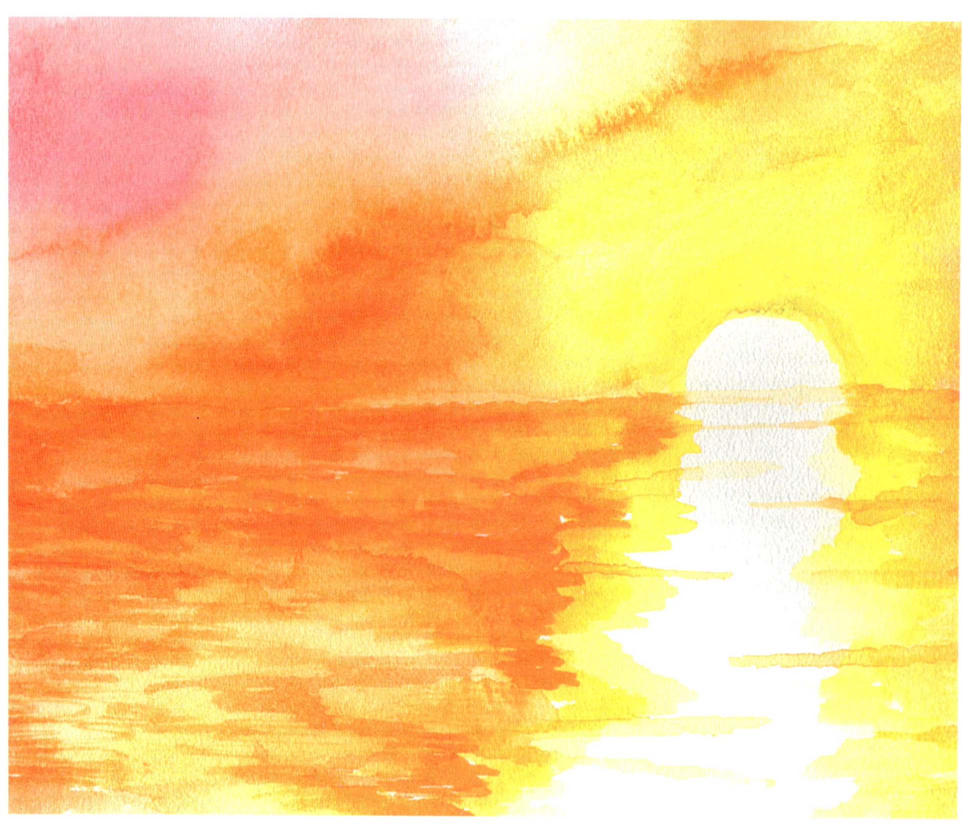

291

A portrait of grief and growth

Try this when
you feel overhwhelmed by emotions after a break-up

You will need
Paper, paint, sponges, foil

20+ minutes

Create an abstract painting using colours to represent all your emotions about a relationship ending. Start by painting a layer with your hands, sponges, or scrunched-up foil that shows the difficult emotions you feel. Then add another layer, using colours to represent positive feelings that can come from letting go of something that was no longer serving you. Notice how they blend to represent your full spectrum of emotions.

SELF-REFLECTION How did the blending of colours represent the complexity of your feelings? What can this painting teach you about embracing the full range of your emotions. You may want to check out emotional management exercises in the previous chapters or talk to an art therapist.

292

Blooming

Try this when
you want to find a way forward

You will need
Pencil, coloured pencils, markers, sticky notes

20+ minutes

The path to overcoming the loss of a relationship is filled with difficult emotions, so it's important to create space for comfort during this time. Draw three different flowers on three sticky notes. In the centre, write down an emotion you want to feel when you have overcome your grief. Inside each petal, write down activities that can bring you closer to that feeling. Place the sticky notes around your home to remind you what to do when you are feeling down.

SELF-REFLECTION Which feeling do you want to experience right now? Can you make time for activities that elicit this feeling in the near future? Can you schedule time this week for one of the activities you wrote down?

Better communication

Communication effectively takes practice. We all have different ways of communicating: some of us are direct, while others might prefer a more amiable approach. For the next four exercises, find a partner to make art with and explore your own communication style.

Try this when
you want to improve the way you communicate with others

40 minutes

293 Create through verbal communication

You will need
Paper, markers, timer

Invite someone you trust to work through these exercises. Set a timer for 5 minutes. Then, create a collaborative piece of art where you both draw something together on the same page. You are allowed to talk to each other.

294 Create through non-verbal communication

You will need
Paper, markers, timer

Now, create another piece of art together. Set the timer for 5 minutes. This time, you will not be allowed to speak to each other, so you must find other ways of communicating in order to work collaboratively.

295 **Share using verbal communication**

You will need
Paper, markers

If you feel verbal communication works best for you, test it here. Draw how you feel right now and share it with the person you have been working with. Show them your artwork and talk about the meaning. Ask the person to draw a response to what you said, then share what their art means with you. You can discuss how that exchange feels for both of you.

296 **Share using non-verbal communication**

You will need
Paper, markers

If non-verbal communication feels more effective, try out this exercise. Draw how you currently feel, then show this to your creative partner in silence. Allow them to draw a response and show it to you without talking. Continue to each draw feelings and responses until you both feel satisfied. If you like, you may then verbally share how this experience felt for both of you.

SELF-REFLECTION Was it easy or hard to create art collaboratively? Did you enjoy it? Can you identify whether your communication preference inclines more towards the verbal or non-verbal? How can you use this information to improve your communication with those around you? How did it feel to share your feelings visually? Did this help enhance the communication with your creative partner? How can visual language improve your relationships in the future?

297

A space for farewell

Try this when
you are ready to let go
of a past relationship

You will need
Found objects, pen, paper

50+ minutes

When a relationship ends, we cannot erase the past, but we can transform how we hold on to it. Collect objects from around your house that evoke both good and bad memories of your past relationship, then arrange them in front of you. Use these as inspiration to write a note, poem, or letter reflecting on your relationship, think about what you gained, what hurt you, and what shaped you. Observe your creation and let any emotions you feel surface. Light a candle or play music if it helps you connect with the moment. When you are ready to say goodbye, donate, remove, or discard the objects in a meaningful way, such as giving them to charity or repurposing them into new artwork.

SELF-REFLECTION What part of this process felt the most tender for you and why? How was it to hold both love and pain in this final farewell? Does letting go of the objects help make space for new things in your life?

298

Better times ahead

Try this when
you are ready to imagine
a happier future

You will need
Paper, pencil, watercolours,
paintbrushes

20+ minutes

Create a landscape that shows how the future might look after a relationship has ended. Include elements that represent your hopes, dreams, needs, and spaces for freedom and healing. Use bridges, paths, weather, or seasons to represent this world.

SELF-REFLECTION What details stand out most in your landscape? Is there a sense of peace, hope, or uncertainty in this future? Are there obstacles or challenges visible in the scene? Did creating this vision change how you feel about moving forward?

299

Nurture the circle

Try this when
you want to nurture
your relationships

You will need
Your favourite art materials, card
cut to the size of a postcard

30 minutes

Relationships aren't just a status, they
are like a living being that needs to be
nurtured to be kept alive and well. Write
a list of people who are special to you,
then create a postcard of appreciation for
every one of them. Send or deliver them
personally to show them that you care.

SELF-REFLECTION Who made it on to your
list, and why were they there? Are these
relationships that you constantly nurture?
Do you ever neglect these relationships?
If so, then try to make more time for
nurturing them.

300

Making others happy
makes us happy

Try this when
you want to feel more
connected with others

You will need
Your favourite art materials, paper
cut to the size of business cards

30 minutes

Feeling connected to those around you
helps protect your mental health. Draw a
tiny artwork, then on the back, write some
encouraging words. Place the artworks
somewhere where people can find them:
maybe on someone's desk, inside a
library book, or on public bulletin boards.
You never know who might discover your
message and find the encouragement
they were looking for.

SELF-REFLECTION Did this experience help
build a sense of belonging to the wider
community around you, or do you feel
you need direct contact with others to
feel truly connected? How did it feel to
make art for others anonymously? Have
you ever found tiny artworks around you
that have helped inspire you?

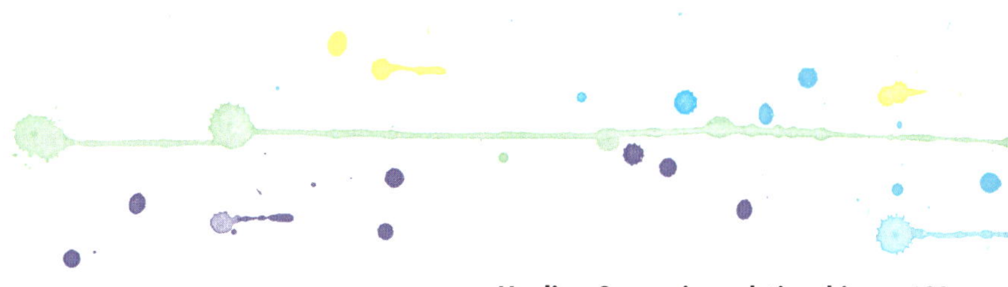

301
Creating connections

Try this when
you need a reminder of
your support system

You will need
Paper, watercolours,
paintbrushes

30+ minutes

Identify people who you feel close to from different
spheres of your life. It might be friends, family, and
people from work or school. If possible, ask each of
them to paint in a small portion of a piece of paper
with a colour of their choosing. If they live far away,
you can ask them what colour and where on the
page they want to be represented and you can paint
it yourself. When you're done, place it somewhere
obvious to remind you that you are not alone.

SELF-REFLECTION Did this experience help build a
sense of belonging to the wider community around
you, or do you feel that you need direct contact with
others to feel truly connected?

302
Part of the art community

Try this when
you want to connect with
like-minded people

You will need
Access to an art event,
notepad, coloured pencils

30+ minutes

Search for art shows that exhibit your favourite art
technique or one that you are curious about, and
attend the event. Before entering, take a moment for
a brief emotional check-in with your coloured pencils
and notepad to express how you're feeling. Enjoy
your visit with curiosity and openness. Notice the
people around you – are they similar to you or
different? Observe the artists' work through a lens
of connection: do they express themselves as you
do? Can you find common ground with others
while experiencing the art? Before leaving, do
another emotional check-in. How do you feel now?

SELF-REFLECTION How did it feel to experience art
connected to your own artistic style? Did you find
commonalities that made you feel understood and
less alone? How can attending art events help us
feel more connected in our experiences?

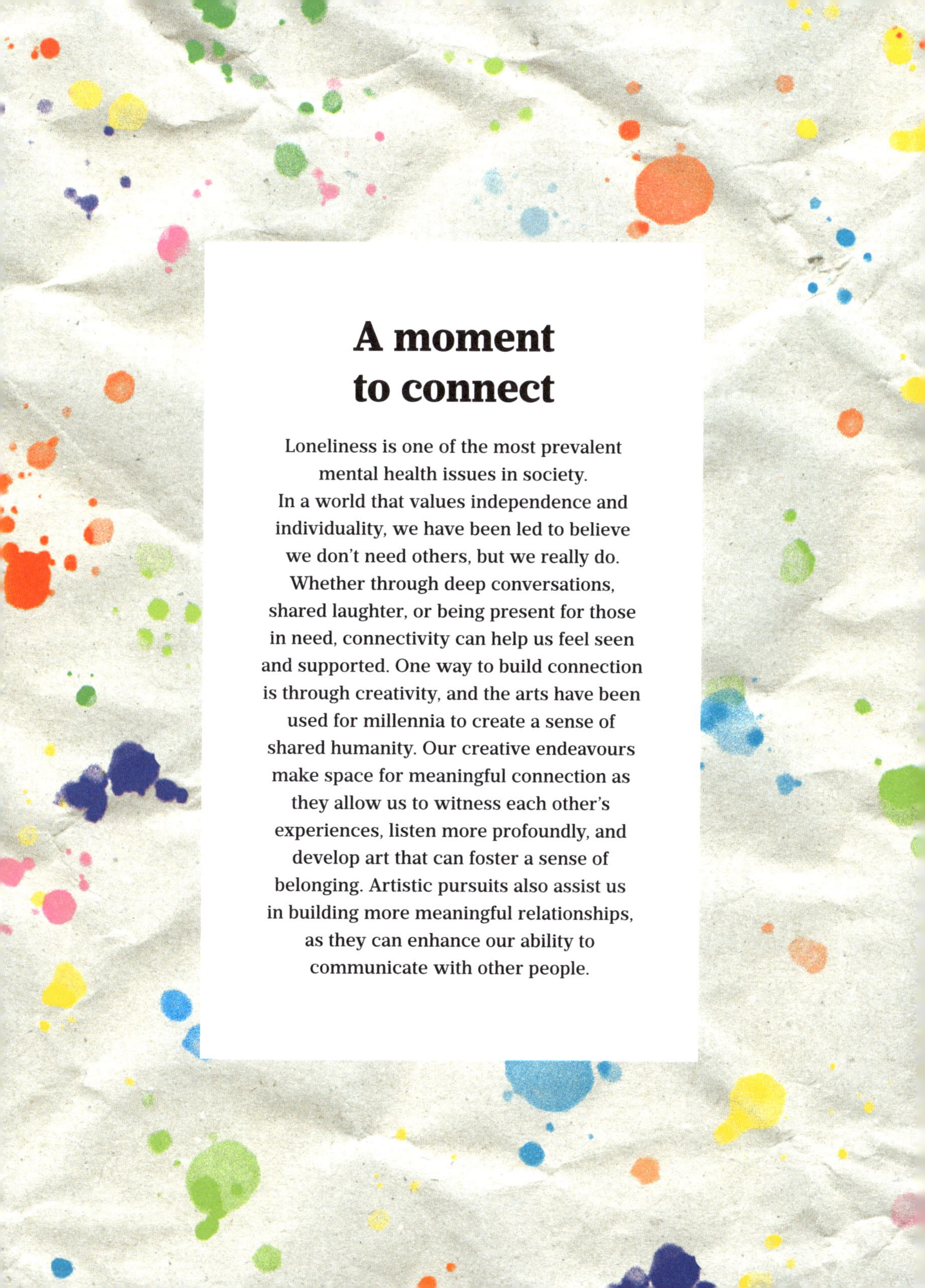

A moment to connect

Loneliness is one of the most prevalent mental health issues in society. In a world that values independence and individuality, we have been led to believe we don't need others, but we really do. Whether through deep conversations, shared laughter, or being present for those in need, connectivity can help us feel seen and supported. One way to build connection is through creativity, and the arts have been used for millennia to create a sense of shared humanity. Our creative endeavours make space for meaningful connection as they allow us to witness each other's experiences, listen more profoundly, and develop art that can foster a sense of belonging. Artistic pursuits also assist us in building more meaningful relationships, as they can enhance our ability to communicate with other people.

303

Building a creative circle part 1

Try this when
you want to experience
a sense of belonging

You will need
Access to a local art event

30+ minutes

Sign up for a local art event that aligns
with your favourite art technique and
allows you to create with others. It can be
an ongoing class or a single workshop.
Notice how creating your art in the
company of others makes you feel.

SELF-REFLECTION How did it feel to
connect with people who share the
same artistic preferences? Could this be
something that could help you connect
with like-minded people?

304

Building a creative circle part 2

Try this when
you want to build a
creative community

You will need
Your favourite art materials

30+ minutes

Creating art in a community builds
stronger bonds. Invite three or more
people you feel comfortable with to your
home, a park, or a place where you feel
it's okay to gather. Remember to clean
up afterwards if it's a public space. You
can all do the same project together, or
everyone can bring the art or craft they
feel comfortable with. Make some tea
and enjoy your creative time together.

SELF-REFLECTION How did it feel to make
art in a group? Was everyone silent, or
was there conversation while creating?
Was this comfortable for you? Could this
be something you do more often?

305

Building a creative circle part 3

Try this when
you want to bring people together through art

You will need
Sketchbook or journal with blank pages, your favourite art materials

30+ minutes

Begin a collaborative art journal that rotates among your family, friends, co-workers, or a group you meet with regularly. Give each person a week to fill a page with colours, drawings, photos, inspiring quotes, or reflections before passing it on. Together you can decide on a theme for each round of creating, or simply let it run its course with no expectations. This can help to foster a sense of connection among group members and create a space for collective expression.

SELF-REFLECTION What purpose could this project serve for you? Is there something you would like to see happen with it? Share your expectations with others, as well as some creative rules to help others and yourself feel safe. Decide how you all feel about sharing the journal with people outside the group, and how to protect everyone's privacy. How long do you want this journal to be worked on? Is it a month, or do you want it to be an annual project? What would happen if someone doesn't follow the time limits and pass the journal on?

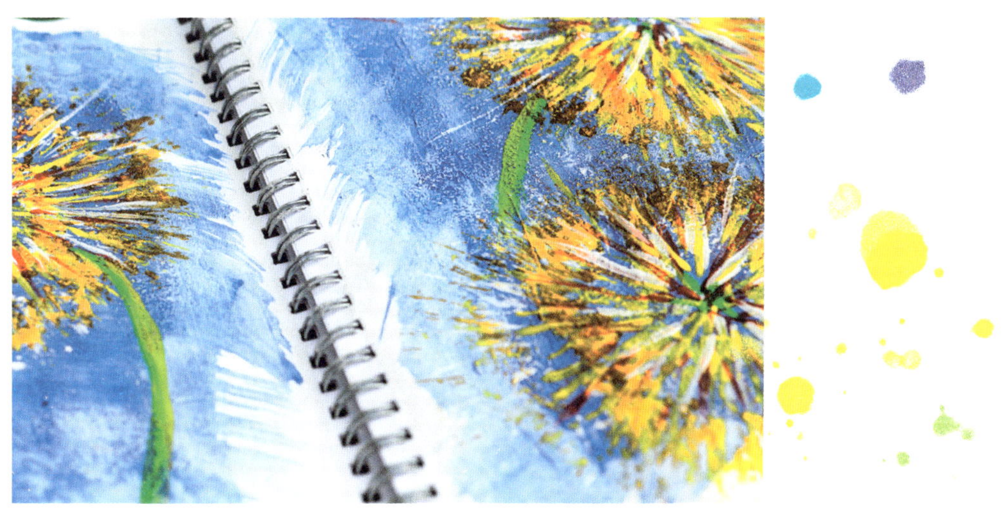

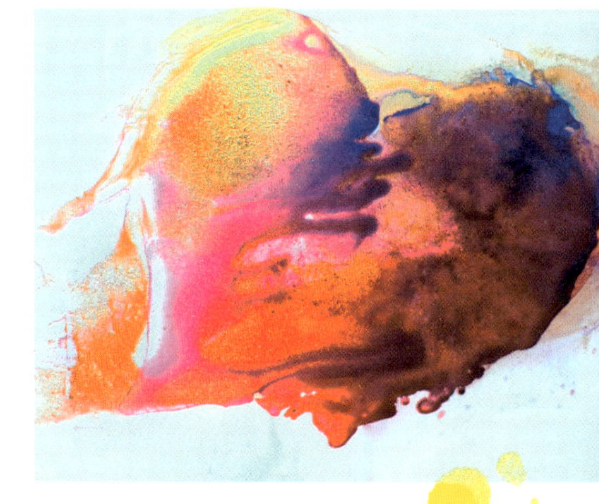

Harnessing self-compassion

Self-compassion means treating ourselves with the same love and kindness we offer others. It isn't about pity, it is about recognizing our shared struggles and using this understanding to help us move forward. Creativity provides a safe space to check in with and nurture ourselves with compassionate intention.

306

Self-compassion 101

Try this when
you feel self-critical

You will need
Paper, markers,
coloured pencils

20 minutes

Fold a piece of paper in half. On one side, draw five thought bubbles, then write a thought you often have when you fail inside each one. On the other side, draw five speech bubbles, and write what you would say to a friend who's dealing with failure in each. Take a moment to notice the difference between how you speak to others and how you speak to yourself. Are you less critical and more encouraging when talking to others?

SELF-REFLECTION How did it feel to observe the way you speak to yourself? Do you think it is easier to be kinder to others? Will it be easy or hard to start using more compassionate language with yourself? Why?

307

Kindness letter

Try this when
you are in need of
self-forgiveness

You will need
Paper, watercolours,
paintbrushes, pen

30 minutes

Paint a piece of paper with colours that feel calming to you. While it's drying, think of a time when you made a mistake. Use the painted page to write a letter to that version of you, sending encouragement and understanding. You can also decorate the paper with symbols that represent self-forgiveness and self-love, such as butterflies, hearts, or interconnected circles.

SELF-REFLECTION Did writing kind words to yourself make you feel uncomfortable? Is it hard to be understanding and forgiving with yourself? Could this mean you are too hard on yourself?

Caring for your inner child

Try this when
you notice negative
self-talk creeping in

You will need
Paper, photo of you as a
child, glue, coloured pencils

30 minutes

Would you dare speak to a child the way you speak to yourself? Glue your childhood photo onto a piece of paper, or use it as inspiration to draw a portrait. Around the image, write words you wish had been said to you when you were small. Shower your inner child with encouragement, showing love and support. You can decorate the page with favourite characters, food, and toys.

SELF-REFLECTION How did it feel to give love and support to your inner child? Could the words you chose have changed your childhood experience if you had heard them? Might they have helped you become a better adult? Next time you are talking down to yourself, remember you are doing it to that same child on the page.

A safe space for your inner child

Try this when
you need to care
for your inner child

You will need
Photo of you as a child, items from
your house, phone camera

20+ minutes

Using objects from around your house, such as a soft blanket, jumper, or scarf, create a nest where your inner child can rest and feel protected. Include cosy textures, soothing colours, or things your inner child would have loved. Place your childhood picture inside the nest and take a photo. Observe how it feels to see yourself held like this. Can you wear or keep the elements that built the nest close to you as a reminder?

SELF-REFLECTION Were you ever held like this as a child? Are the clothing items you chose things you wear often? Can you treat yourself with softness, or does that make you feel uncomfortable?

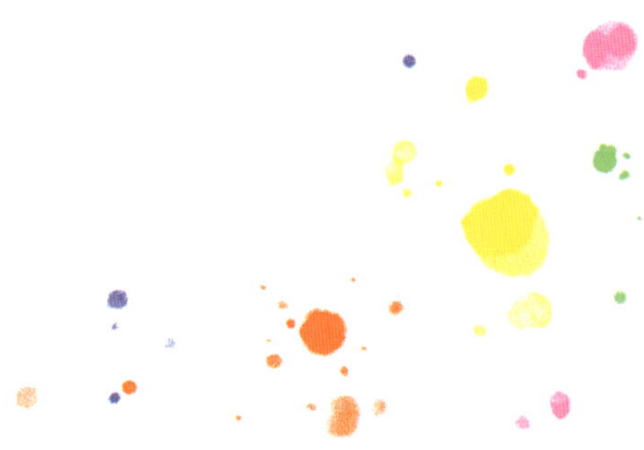

310

Caring for your inner adolescent

Try this when
you feel misunderstood

You will need
Paper, photo of you as a teenager, glue, coloured pencils

30 minutes

What would you tell your angsty adolescent self that could help soothe them? Glue a photo of you as a teenager onto a piece of paper, or draw it. Around the image, write words you wish had been said to you when you were feeling misunderstood. Shower this adolescent with empathy and guidance. You can also decorate the page with their favourite films, bands, food, or books.

SELF-REFLECTION How did it feel to reconnect with your inner adolescent? Was it healing to receive words of support? Would your teenage self be proud of who you have become?

311

A gift for my teenage self

Try this when
you want to connect with your teenage self

You will need
Paper, coloured pencils, markers

30 minutes

Create an album cover for a soundtrack representing you as a teenager. It should capture your energy and predominant emotions at that moment in time. On the back, write a playlist of the songs that would be included. Then, write down what that version of you needed the most.

SELF-REFLECTION How do you feel giving space for your teenage self to emerge? What was it like to connect with your teenage energy? Is it comfortable to hold that part of yourself with compassion and love? If you could go back in time, what would you tell yourself?

312

All I want

Try this when
you're ready to give yourself the care you deserve

You will need
Paper, pencil, markers, coloured pencils

20 minutes

Draw or print out a blank human figure, then draw or write the answers to the following questions: what do you need physically? What do you need mentally? What do you need emotionally? What do you need from your relationships? What do you need spiritually?

SELF-REFLECTION Have you been satisfying all of your different needs, or do you favour some over others? What needs do you usually prioritize? Could you start including others you haven't paid attention to in order to become more balanced?

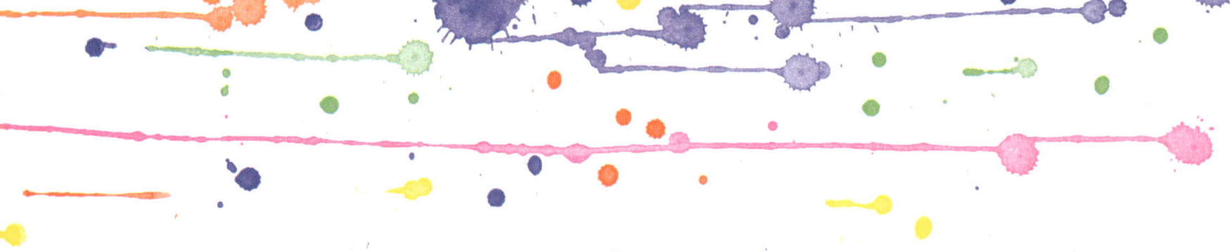

313

Taking care of me

Try this when
you need to remember that
your wellbeing matters

You will need
Paper, pencil, markers,
coloured pencils,
watercolours, paintbrushes

30 minutes

Draw a medical prescription. On it, write down what helps to soothe you. It can be scents, colours, places, people, or specific activities. Then, write down how much time you need with each of these when you are going through difficult periods. Can you make this a reality? Maybe hang it on your fridge as a reminder.

SELF-REFLECTION Are the things you prescribed easy to give to yourself? Next time you experience failure, could you use these things to afford yourself more compassion? Or do they feel undeserved? If this is the case, remember to hold yourself with kindness.

314

Self-compassion filter

Try this when
you are being too
hard on yourself

You will need
Paper, pen

30 minutes

This exercise can bring up strong emotions, so make sure you're in a positive and safe headspace before you begin. Write down five self-critical thoughts starting with "I", leaving plenty of space between each one – for example, "I'm not good enough" or "I can't do this". Then, imagine hearing these words from a close friend or your inner child. How would you respond? Next, write down your supportive responses as "I" statements to yourself. For example, if your thought is, "I'm not good enough", you might respond, "I am doing my best and I am enough".

SELF-REFLECTION How did it feel to direct the compassion you usually give to others back towards yourself? Did this process help you soften your inner critic? The next time you notice negative self-talk, can you try replacing it with one of these more supportive thoughts?

315

Our common humanity

Try this when
you feel alone in
your struggles

You will need
Paper, coloured pencils,
markers, computer
or phone

20 minutes

Self-compassion stems from recognizing our shared humanity; we are not alone in our struggles. Think of a minor struggle you are experiencing. Do you know anyone close to you who is struggling with the same? Create a postcard for them, letting them know they are not alone, and provide words of encouragement. You don't have to send it. If you can't think of anyone, look online for forums that discuss your issue, then choose one of the testimonials and create a postcard for that person.

SELF-REFLECTION Did you notice how many people share your kind of suffering? Does a shared burden reduce the stress of feeling like the "only one"? Or do you feel guilty about feeling better just because others are suffering too?

316

Our imperfections connect us to others

Try this when
you want to soften
self-judgement

You will need
Pencil, small notepad
or sketchbook

**20+ minutes throughout
the day**

Over the course of a day, notice when others make small mistakes. Choose one situation and draw a rough sketch of it. Try to understand what happened without being critical, and consider why it might have occurred. Could the same thing happen to you? Being mindful of others' shortcomings can remind us that we are all vulnerable.

SELF-REFLECTION How did it feel to view others' mistakes with compassion instead of judgement? Can this shift in perspective help you be kinder to yourself? Can you use this experience to feel less alone?

317

Self-compassion is a two-way street part 1

Try this when
you need to show
yourself more love

You will need
Paper, coloured pencils, markers

20 minutes

Divide a piece of paper into three columns. In the first column, draw things that give you comfort. It might be a blanket, a smell, or a person. In the second column, draw things that soothe you – perhaps a certain type of music, a warm bath, or a hug. In the third, draw what helps you feel validated. How do you show appreciation for yourself? Perhaps you buy a small treat, or give yourself time to nap after a long day.

SELF-REFLECTION Was it easy or hard to identify ways that you can hold yourself more lovingly? How often do you engage in the activities you identified? Can you do some of them more for the next couple of weeks?

318

Self-compassion is a two-way street part 2

Try this when
you're ready to prioritize yourself

You will need
Paper, coloured pencils, markers

20 minutes

Using the paper from the previous exercise, draw three more columns on the back. In the first column, draw things you do to protect yourself. Perhaps you have started setting firmer boundaries, or exercise for your health. In the second column, demonstrate how you provide what you need for yourself. For example, do you plan ahead to give yourself time for enjoyment? In the third, draw what helps you to stay motivated. Do you have a vision board to inspire you? Or do you keep reminders of positive affirmations?

SELF-REFLECTION Do you think you are good at actively looking after yourself? Or is this something you struggle with? Can you start being more proactive about protecting your needs and wants?

319

Compassion may not be working... and that's okay

Try this when
self-compassion feels uncomfortable

You will need
Paper, coloured pencils, markers

15 minutes

Becoming more compassionate towards yourself isn't always easy. Self-compassion means fully accepting yourself, including the parts you may feel less comfortable with. If you feel that a self-compassion practice isn't working for you, try drawing how you feel – whether as a symbol or an abstract image. Validating your emotions can help release the expectation that self-compassion should only make you feel good.

SELF-REFLECTION Could you use your art to hold and acknowledge your discomfort? When self-compassion didn't make you feel better, did you blame yourself? Are you able to accept your uncomfortable feelings without judgement?

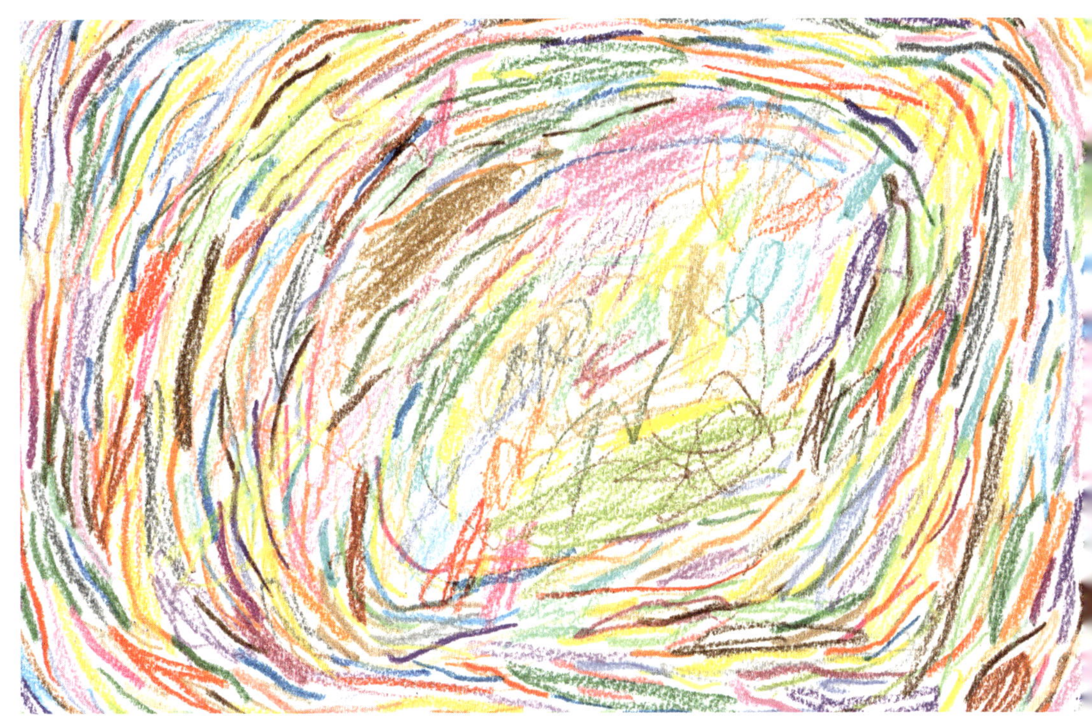

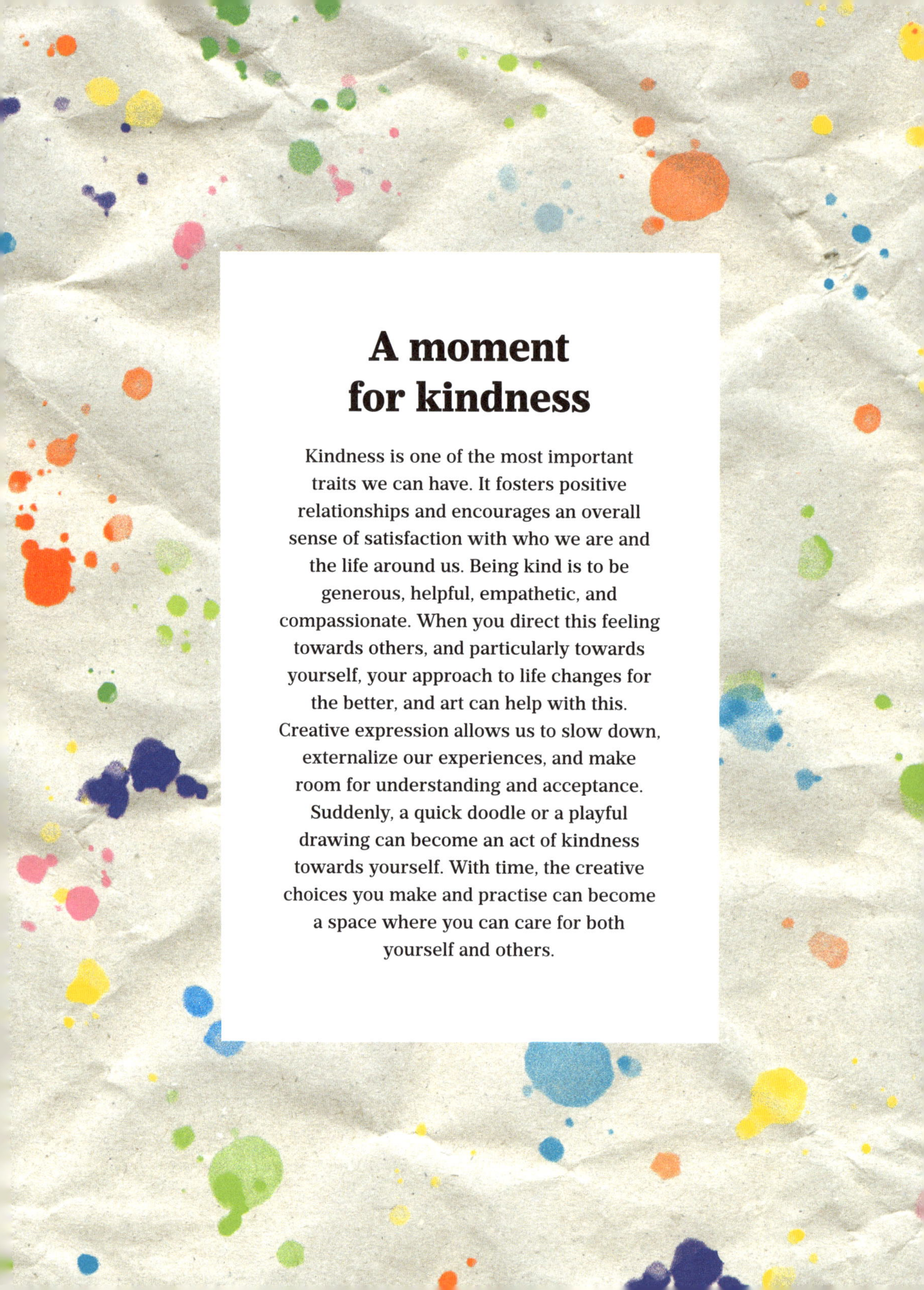

A moment for kindness

Kindness is one of the most important traits we can have. It fosters positive relationships and encourages an overall sense of satisfaction with who we are and the life around us. Being kind is to be generous, helpful, empathetic, and compassionate. When you direct this feeling towards others, and particularly towards yourself, your approach to life changes for the better, and art can help with this. Creative expression allows us to slow down, externalize our experiences, and make room for understanding and acceptance. Suddenly, a quick doodle or a playful drawing can become an act of kindness towards yourself. With time, the creative choices you make and practise can become a space where you can care for both yourself and others.

320

Practising self-acceptance

Try this when
you're ready to embrace
all parts of yourself

You will need
Paper, found object to
represent yourself,
pencil, eraser

20 minutes

Choose an object to represent the things that you love about yourself. Go outside and place the item so that the sun casts its shadow onto your paper, then draw the outline of the shadow with a pencil. Inside the shadow, write down things you judge yourself about the most. They can be feelings you experience, personality traits, or past experiences. Around the shadow, write down the things that you love about yourself. Now erase the outline of the shadow. Can you notice both parts of you co-existing?

SELF-REFLECTION Which side was easier to write about – the loving or the judgemental one? How did it feel to integrate both parts of yourself? What small steps can you take to embrace both your negative and positive sides?

321

Walking the self-compassion path

Try this when
you want to strengthen your
self-compassion habit

You will need
Paper, coloured pencils,
watercolours, paintbrushes

30+ minutes daily

Building self-compassion practice requires time and commitment. Paint a circle the size of your palm to acknowledge a time you were compassionate towards yourself. Add some words or draw what you did on top of the circle. Repeat this exercise every evening for three weeks using the same piece of paper. Over time, colours and circles will start overlapping, and that's fine. Notice how progress isn't linear, but layered and evolving.

SELF-REFLECTION Were you able to do this exercise for 21 days straight? If you couldn't, what got in the way? If you were able to complete the exercise, did you notice any difference in the way you felt compared to when you started your journey?

322

Please forgive me

Try this when
self-blame feels
overwhelming

You will need
Paper, coloured pencils,
markers

20 minutes

Sometimes, it might seem easier to forgive others than to forgive yourself. Think of a small mistake you made and imagine you are being taken to court. Draw a ticket and write down the things you are accusing yourself of. On another piece of paper, write how you would defend this case if you were a lawyer. Were there things you weren't aware of that led to making the mistake? Were you having a bad day? Was there something else to blame, beside yourself, that contributed to the mistake?

SELF-REFLECTION Did you accuse yourself too harshly? Were you able to see the bigger picture and step away from self-blame? What small steps can you take to show yourself more forgiveness?

323

Forgive and learn

Try this when
you are ready to learn
from your mistakes

You will need
Paper, coloured pencils,
markers

20 minutes

When we make a mistake, we want to learn from it and, hopefully, not repeat it. Reflect on a recent mistake you've made. Divide a piece of paper in half. On one side, draw yourself making the mistake. On the other side, illustrate what you could do differently next time to avoid a similar situation, along with the lessons you've learnt.

SELF-REFLECTION Was it helpful to reflect on the lessons learnt from your mistake? Do you think this drawing can support you in avoiding similar mistakes in the future? Can approaching your mistakes creatively help you cultivate more self-forgiveness?

324

Failure vs growth

Try this when
you want to move forward
with a growth mindset

You will need
Paper, coloured
pencils, markers

20 minutes

Fold a piece of paper into three sections. In the first section, draw what failure feels like for you. In the last section, draw what growth feels like. In the middle, write questions you can ask yourself that move you from one space to other. For example: what can I learn from the experience? Can I shift my language or perspective? What is this experience teaching me about myself?

SELF-REFLECTION What are the main differences you notice between your perceptions of failure and growth? Do you feel you lean more towards one or the other? Can having a list of questions help you shift your mindset when you're feeling low?

325

Cup of tea

Try this when
you feel drained

You will need
Paper, coloured pencils,
markers

20 minutes

Draw a cup, then next to it, draw a box containing six different types of tea. Assign an image or words that help you feel nourished and restored next to each tea: perhaps "enjoying a nice meal" or "having an early night". Use this drawing as inspiration when you are in need of showing yourself some loving care.

SELF-REFLECTION How often do you give yourself space to recharge? Are the ideas you drew easy to accomplish? Can you come back to this drawing when you are feeling drained?

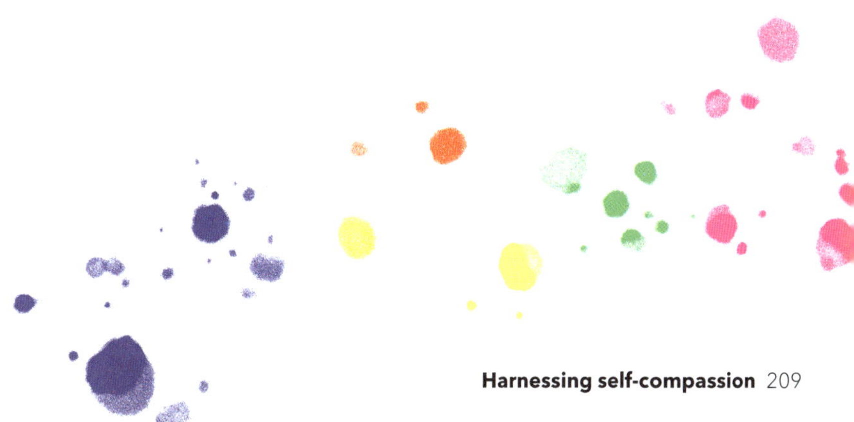

What we learn
from loving kindness

Loving kindness is a meditation used in mindful practice to help build feelings of warmth and compassion towards yourself and others. It stems from Hindu and Buddhist traditions, and is believed to have been taught to help monks overcome adversity. This practice can be used to develop unconditional positive regard as a path towards inner peace.

Try this when
you need to connect to
love and warmth

1 hour 20 minutes

326 **Loving you**

You will need
Paper, coloured
pencils, markers

Think of a person or animal you care for deeply – someone who brings you calm and joy – then draw a portrait of them. It can be a literal representation or abstract. When you have finished, take a moment to wish them well, sending your love, healing energy, and well wishes their way.

327 **Loving me**

You will need
Photo of yourself, pen

Now, turn the same loving energy towards yourself. Set your photo in front of you and send yourself the same good wishes. When you are done meditating, write some words on the back of the photo to remind you of the positive energy you connected with.

328 Loving you is loving me

You will need

Paper, coloured pencils,
markers, phone or computer

There are many loving kindness meditations to be found online that you can use for this exercise. Find one featuring a voice that feels soothing. Listen to it, then create a visual representation of your experience. It could be gentle waves in soft colours, or something representative of loving feelings such as sunflowers or hearts.

329 May I be...

You will need

Paper, coloured pencils,
wmarkers

The phrases used in a loving kindness meditation often begin with "May I", as these words create space for heartfelt wishes. On the top of a page, write a message beginning with "May I" and draw what you wish for yourself. Think of simple phrases such as "be loved authentically", "be safe from harm", and "be accepted for who I am".

SELF-REFLECTION How did it feel to connect with your loved one in the first exercise? Did it generate a positive feeling? Would you be able to communicate these wishes personally, such as by calling or hugging them? What feelings did you experience while meditating? How did it feel to send yourself the same positive energy you sent to someone else? Was it easy or difficult to find wishes for yourself? Can you take a moment to put your hand on your chest and whisper them to yourself?

330

Things you are great at

Try this when
you want to celebrate
who you are

You will need
Paper, coloured pencils, pen

30 minutes

There are positive things about yourself that make you, *you*. Draw an oval almost the size of the paper. Inside it, draw curved lines that become smaller, emulating the whorls of a fingerprint. Look at your own fingerprint for inspiration. Leave enough space between the lines to write between them. Then, write the things that make you great inside the fingerprint, starting every line with "I am". Perhaps you are altruistic, empathic, or thoughtful? Maybe you have wonderful passions. Change colours for different phrases. If you have a hard time identifying these things, think about what you are usually recognized for, or ask loved ones what they like about you. What do they think makes up the essence of you?

SELF-REFLECTION Do you think there are things you were born with that make you special, or did you learn to become the way you are? How does it feel to be recognized for your positive attributes? Were you surprised by the things people shared with you, or did you know them already?

331

Take yourself on a date

Try this when
you need to make
time for you

You will need
Small notebook or
sketchbook, coloured pencils

30+ minutes

Taking yourself on a solo date can help you better understand and build a deeper connection with yourself. Look for an art or cultural exhibition that interests you and set a date to attend it. While you are there, document it by sketching out things that intrigue you or catch your attention. At the end, buy yourself a drink and sit down to reflect on the experience. Think about how it might reflect who you are, whether it offered new ideas or insights about yourself, or if it transformed you in any way.

SELF-REFLECTION Could you use this date to get to know yourself better? Were you able to connect more meaningfully with yourself? If you were to take yourself out on a second date, where would you go?

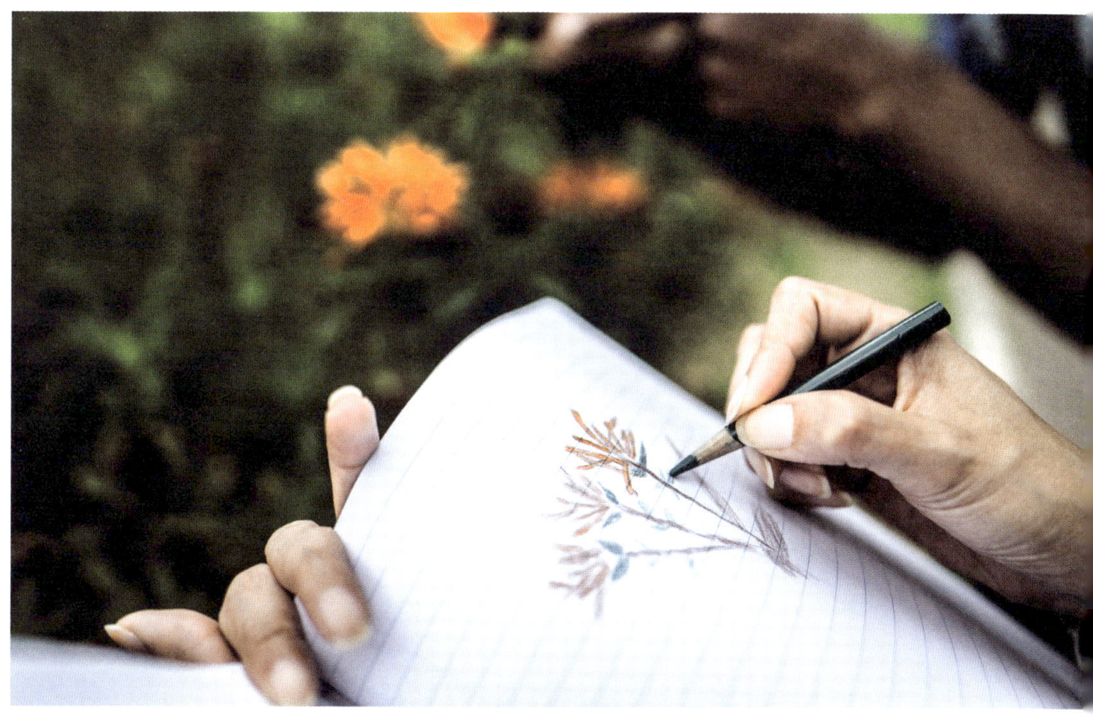

332

Buy yourself flowers

Try this when
your cup feels empty

You will need
Paper, markers,
coloured pencils

30 minutes

Draw a floral bouquet just for you, filled with your favourite flowers. Then, assign an act of love you can show yourself to each flower. What do you do for yourself? Maybe it's cooking, caring for your home, or getting yourself to your art therapy session.
How do you engage in physical touch? It could be taking a hot shower, or wearing soft clothing. Do you give yourself words of affirmation, such as positive self-talk or journalling? Do you schedule any quality time for yourself, or give yourself gifts?

SELF-REFLECTION Think about how you show your love for others. Do you give yourself love in the same way? Do you find it easier to receive love from yourself or from others?

Loving me, lifting us

Try this when
you want to share
small acts of kindness

You will need
Paper, favourite
art materials

20 minutes

Serving others can not only help those around you, but also help you feel good. Divide a piece of paper into eight squares. Inside each, draw something that depicts a healthy, connected community. It could be walking a neighbour's dog, a thriving community garden, or a street party. On the back of each square, write down one thing you can contribute to make this vision real. Perhaps organizing an outing with neighbours who you notice are lonely? Making a difference doesn't need to be a huge act of self-sacrifice – it can also be achieved through small actions.

SELF-REFLECTION What is your attitude towards public service? Do you believe you can make a difference to other people's lives? Can you notice how you can use your attributes to help make the world a better place for others?

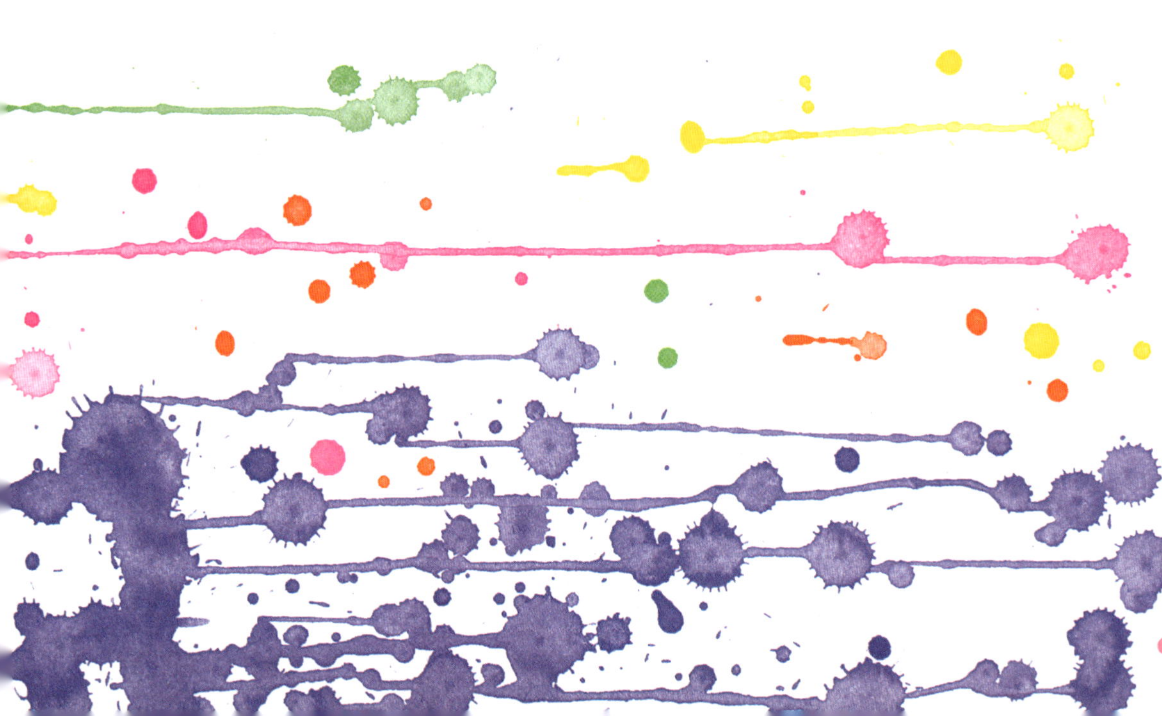

334

Helping hands

Try this when
you want to recognize your
power to make a difference

You will need
Paper, coloured pencils,
markers, tape

20 minutes

Tape two pieces of paper together so you have a
large surface to work on, then trace both your hands,
one on each page. Inside the outlines, write or draw
ways in which you can help others or improve your
community. It can be small things like picking up
rubbish, offering emotional support to a friend, or
looking for volunteer opportunities to improve the
local area.

SELF-REFLECTION How did it feel to think about
yourself as an agent of change? Are there things you
are already doing? Do you take time to acknowledge
the good you do for the world?

335

The portrait of a
world-changer

Try this when
you are ready to share
your gifts with the world

You will need
Paper, photo of yourself,
markers, paint,
paintbrushes, glue

20 minutes

Cut out your face from a photo and paste it onto
a piece of paper. Think of your talents, and how
you can use them for the greater good. Now draw
a portrait that depicts you as an agent of change,
including images that show how you use your
strengths to help others. Maybe you are a good
listener and volunteer for a charity. Or you might
be great at voicing your opinions and have become
an advocate for a cause you believe in. How about
using your superior cooking skills and volunteering
at a soup kitchen?

SELF-REFLECTION Was it easy to identify and connect
with your strengths? How does it feel to notice how
much you can do for your community? Do you
believe in your ability to change the world?

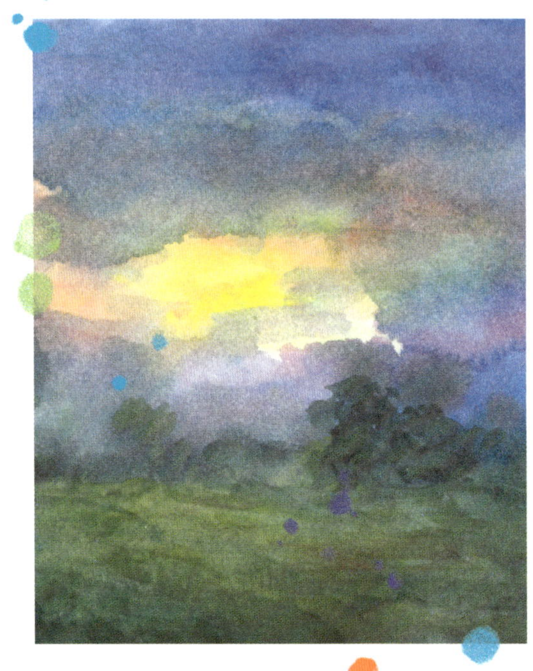

Expressing gratitude

Being grateful can help foster a sense of fulfilment and connection, highlighting the value of community and strengthening social bonds. However, gratitude is also complex, and if forced, it can feel pressured and keep you stuck in negative patterns. Art can help us transform thankfulness into something tangible, boosting our mood, reducing stress, and strengthening our relationships.

336

I am alive!

Try this when
you want to notice the
beauty around you

You will need
Small notepad or
sketchbook, pencil,
coloured pencils

20+ minutes

Go for a walk outside, preferably in nature. Then,
tuning in to your senses, draw something you notice
that's pleasurable. Maybe you can see beauty around
you, or feel the warmth of the sun on your skin.
Perhaps there's music playing somewhere, or you can
smell fresh air or flowers. When you finish, take time
to feel grateful for being able to savour this moment.

SELF-REFLECTION How did it feel to use your body to
connect with positive experiences around you? Do
you take your body's abilities for granted? Can you
integrate this small connectivity practice into your life
as you go about your day?

337

Acknowledging
the big things

Try this when
you want to deepen your
sense of gratitude

You will need
Small notepad or
sketchbook, pencil,
coloured pencils

10+ minute sessions

When life is stressful, we might lose sight of all the
good things that are happening around us. Take a
moment to recognize the big things you can count
on to have a comfortable life. Take a full day to weave
in and out of this activity and sketch the things that
make your life easy. For example, maybe you enjoy
good health, a supportive family, or are part of a
tight-knit community.

SELF-REFLECTION How many things were you able to
observe in one day? Do you feel you take them for
granted? Would you like to keep adding more to the
list and extend this practice for three days or a week?
This approach allows you to engage with the practice
intermittently, making it more manageable and
integrated into your daily routine.

338
Acknowledging the small things

Try this when
you want to appreciate the simple things that make life easier

You will need
Small notepad or sketchbook, pencil, coloured pencils

10+ minute sessions

It's often said that, even though the big things in life matter, it is in the details where we can benefit from gratitude most. Spend a day weaving in and out of this activity, drawing the things you've done to make your life more comfortable. Perhaps you've bought cosy shoes, made time to connect with good friends, or created a peaceful space at home.

SELF-REFLECTION How well have you been able to provide for youself? Do you feel proud about this, or do you take it for granted? Remember that celebrating your wins can help your sense of self-worth. Would you like to extend this practice for three days or even a week?

339
Tree of support

Try this when
you want to understand how privilege has impacted your life

You will need
Paper, pencil, coloured pencils, markers

20+ minutes

Privilege doesn't mean you haven't worked hard or aren't familiar with struggles. It simply acknowledges that there are certain obstacles you don't have to face in life. Draw a tree with deep roots and robust branches. Around the roots, write down things that have quietly supported you, such as a stable home, financial security, or access to education. Use the branches to write down ways you can use these as a platform to support others. Can you help someone in need?

SELF-REFLECTION Do conversations about privilege make you feel guilty or grateful? How can you extend your good fortune to help others? How do you become the difference you want to see in the world?

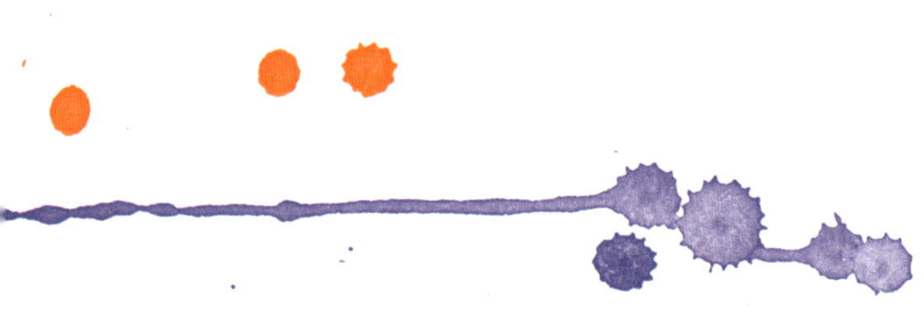

340

Shine on

Try this when
you want to build
a daily gratitude habit

You will need
Paper, coloured pencils

5 minutes daily

In the centre of a sheet of paper, draw a sun with seven rays of sunshine extending from it. Over the course of a week, write down something you are grateful for on a different ray.

SELF-REFLECTION How did it feel to have a daily gratitude practice? Did you notice a shift in your mood? What themes or similarities do you see in your gratitude list?

341

Gratitude ladder

Try this when
you want to recognize those
who support you

You will need
Paper, markers

15 minutes

Draw a ladder, then on each rung or next to it, write the name of a person who you consider a mentor or guide that you want to thank for having lifted you up or helped you overcome a difficult time.

SELF-REFLECTION Are the people who have helped you still a part of your life? Have you let them know what they have done for you? Do you share your gratitude with others openly?

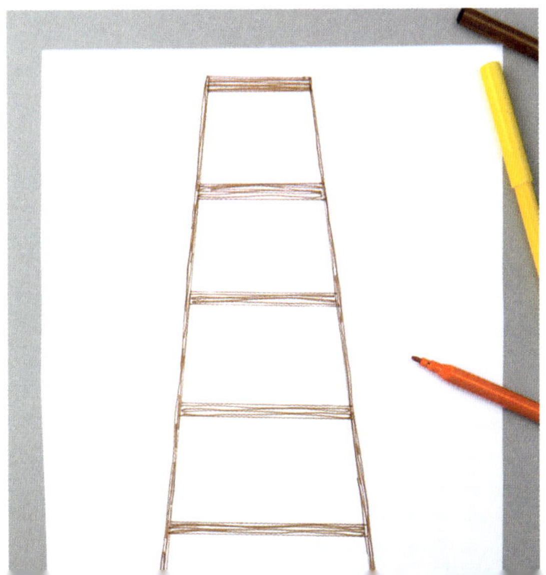

342

Gratitude chain

Try this when
you want to brighten your days with simple moments of gratitude

You will need
21 strips of paper, stapler, pen

10 minutes daily

Every day for three weeks, write down something or someone you are grateful for on a strip of paper. Then, fold it into a loop and staple it together to slowly form a paper chain. Keep this somewhere visible as a reminder of all the good things you have in your life.

SELF-REFLECTION Were you able to complete 21 gratitude notes over 21 consecutive days? If you weren't, what got in the way? Can creative projects help you deepen your gratitude practice?

343

Hands that hold me

Try this when
you want to celebrate the people who support you

You will need
Paper, favourite art materials

30 minutes

Trace your hand five times, slightly overlapping each tracing so they connect with one another. Label each hand with the name of a person you are grateful for and decorate it by illustrating what they bring to your life – maybe good advice or a shoulder to cry on.

SELF-REFLECTION How do these people help support your mental health? Are there ways you can show them your gratitude? What is the most important thing anyone has given you in your life?

344
Small shift

Try this when
you need a reminder of what's
already good in your life

You will need
Found objects, paper, pen

20+ minutes

Whenever you start to ruminate on the
things that are still missing from your life,
walk around your home and find five
objects that remind you of something
you are grateful to have accomplished.
Perhaps it's a souvenir from a trip you
worked hard for, something you made,
or a family photo. Choose one that feels
the most important to you and write
down how this object can serve as a
reminder that even though you might
not have everything, you do currently
have – and are – enough.

SELF-REFLECTION Was it hard to stop
thinking about what is missing and
identify things to be thankful for in your
life? Could this be a sign of a need to
slow down and be more present instead
of future focused?

345
Appreciation for the body

Try this when
you need to treat your body
with more kindness

You will need
Non-toxic watercolours,
paintbrushes, eyeliner

20+ minutes

Our bodies do so much for us, and
we rarely pause to thank them. Take a
moment to draw hearts on different
parts of your body, thanking that body
part for what it does for you. For example,
thank your lungs for breathing and
keeping you alive.

SELF-REFLECTION How did it feel to show
gratitude towards your body? Can having
more gratitude for your body improve
your sense of self-compassion? Are there
any changes you can implement in your
lifestyle to show gratitude for what your
body does for you?

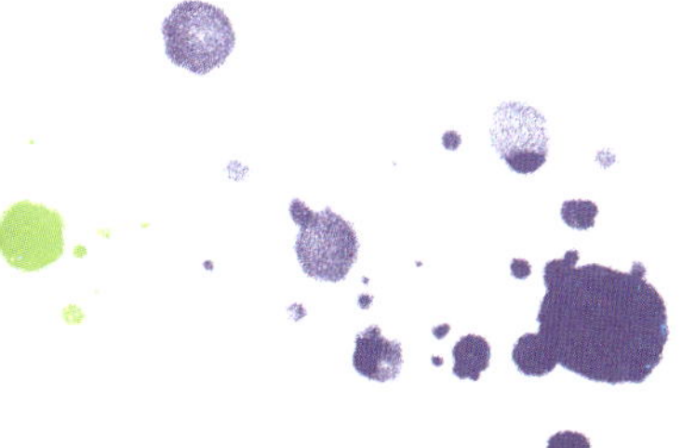

346

Appreciation for the environment

Try this when
you want to reconnect with the natural world

You will need
Paper, watercolours, paintbrushes, coloured pencils

20+ minutes

Connect to the natural world by thinking of something in nature that you find comforting. It can be a spot in the park, the beach, mountains, or a plant in your home. Imagine how it looks, smells, sounds, or the feeling that it creates within you. Then, paint a representation of that place or thing, and write down three things you are grateful for that nature provides. You can also add how you will take care of the environment to show your appreciation for it.

SELF-REFLECTION When was the last time you intentionally connected with nature? What does nature provide for you emotionally? How can we give gratitude for these benefits to our wellbeing?

347

Appreciation for creativity

Try this when
you want to connect with the beauty of art

You will need
Paper, markers, computer or phone

15 minutes

Look around your home or online for the following: your favourite song, painting, poem, and film. Take a moment to sit with how each of these pieces of art makes you feel, holding it and its creator in gratitude for existing.

SELF-REFLECTION What have these art pieces contributed to your life? Can you imagine your life without them? How does it feel to show gratitude for an object or creation and not something sentient?

348

Appreciation for your culture

Try this when
you want to celebrate
your culture

You will need
Found objects, phone
or computer

20+ minutes

Find seven objects around your home that represent your cultural background. They can be family heirlooms, foods or spices, or decorative objects. If you don't have anything specific, look online for representations of your culture(s). Take a moment to be grateful for your heritage. Notice how your culture has given you strengths and things to be proud of.

SELF-REFLECTION Are there parts of your cultural heritage that you are most proud of? Are there things about it that you don't like? Are there any parts of your heritage you didn't like before but now count as a blessing?

349

Appreciation for the unknown

Try this when
you want to build trust
in the unknown

You will need
Paper, coloured pencils,
watercolours, paintbrushes

15 minutes

Paint a picture of a starry night. While it dries, think of at least five moments when you experienced an unexpected blessing – like running late but finding no traffic. Then, choose five stars and paint a small symbol next to each to represent why you felt grateful. Was it for your good fortune, or for feeling protected by something bigger than yourself?

SELF-REFLECTION Do you notice these little magic moments in your life and feel gratitude for them? Can they serve as reminders that not everything is lost and that good things can happen unexpectedly? Can they be a reminder to let go of control and have more trust in your life's journey?

350

The gift

Try this when
you want to reflect on what
life has given you

You will need
Paper, favourite art materials

20+ minutes

Draw an open gift box containing representations of things that have helped you in life and nurtured personal growth. It could be emotional support, special opportunities, or memorable personal events. Place your hand on your chest and connect with the emotion this gift evokes.

SELF-REFLECTION Was this gift a single event in your life, or is this something you receive continually? Have you shown gratitude for this gift directly? How did it feel to connect with this appreciative feeling?

351

Gratitude reminder

Try this when
you feel overwhelmed
by negativity

You will need
Paper, coloured pencils,
black marker

20+ minutes

Use a black marker to doodle on a piece of paper – the more intersections and circles the better. Then, choose different colours to represent yourself, the people around you, creativity, nature, and home. Colour in some of the blank spaces created by the doodle and place the finished piece somewhere you can see it. At least once a week, use this art as a prompt to give gratitude for each of those things. For example, you might be grateful to be home after a tough day.

SELF-REFLECTION Can setting a specific time for this reflective moment help you integrate a gratitude practice into your daily life? How can having daily or recurring moments of gratitude help shift your mood and affect? Could you add other concepts to your creation, such as work, school, pets, or community?

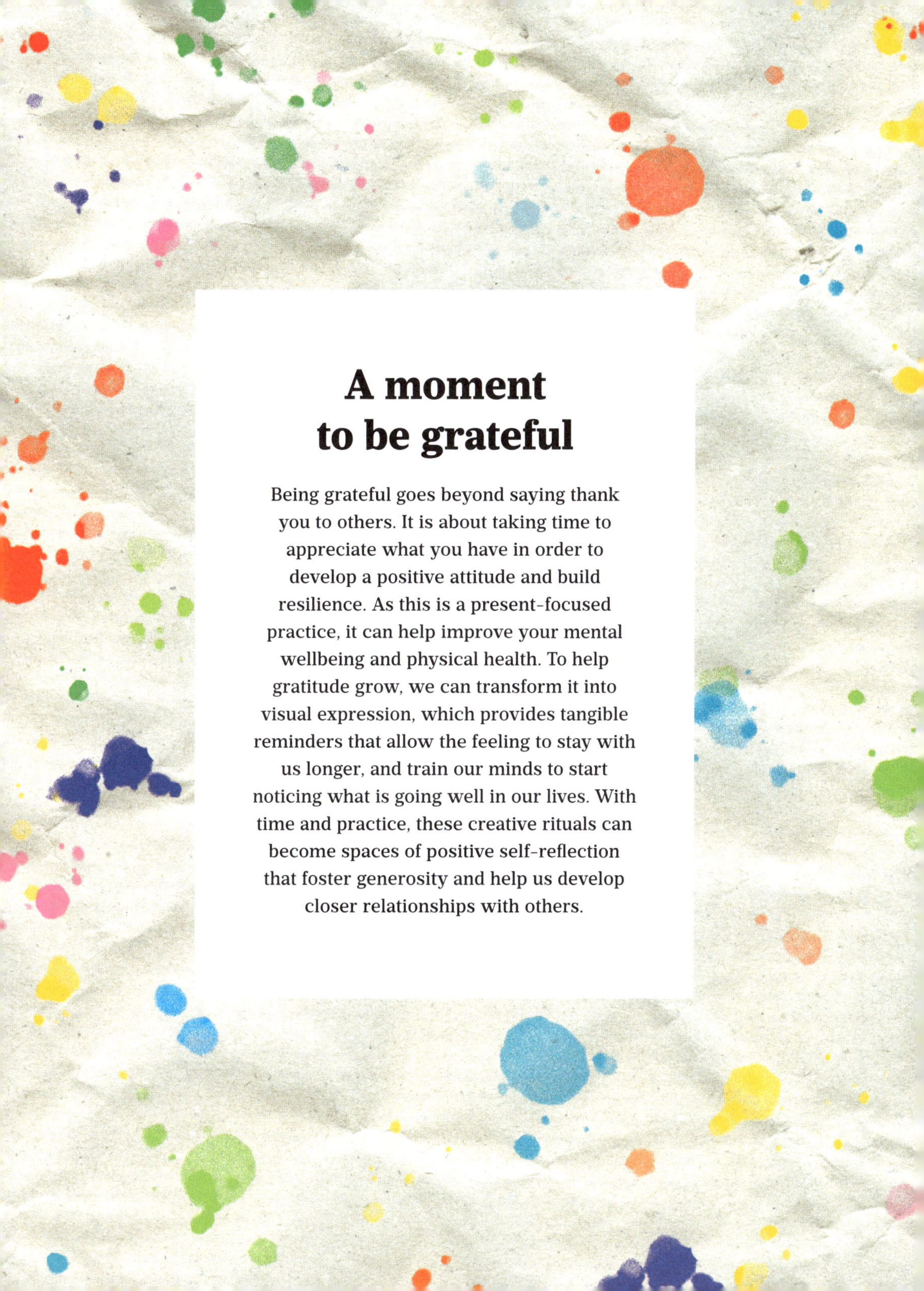

A moment to be grateful

Being grateful goes beyond saying thank you to others. It is about taking time to appreciate what you have in order to develop a positive attitude and build resilience. As this is a present-focused practice, it can help improve your mental wellbeing and physical health. To help gratitude grow, we can transform it into visual expression, which provides tangible reminders that allow the feeling to stay with us longer, and train our minds to start noticing what is going well in our lives. With time and practice, these creative rituals can become spaces of positive self-reflection that foster generosity and help us develop closer relationships with others.

352

The rock and the ripple part 1

Try this when
you feel weighed down

You will need
Rock, paint, paintbrushes

20+ minutes

Paint a rock with colours that represent gratitude for you. Whenever you are feeling down, hold this rock and think about a moment or a person that transformed your day or even your life. It may be a stranger who helped you when you were in distress, or a good teacher who inspired you. Use the rock's weight to help ground you in knowing that through struggles, positive moments can have more weight.

SELF-REFLECTION Could you easily identify a moment or person who helped you? Do positive moments carry more weight for you? Or do you tend to focus on the negative?

353

The rock and the ripple part 2

Try this when
you want to spread kindness

You will need
Paper, rock, paint, paintbrushes

20+ minutes

Place the rock from the previous exercise in the middle of a piece of paper and paint circles around it, mimicking the ripples when a rock falls into water. Think about how the kindness you receive can motivate you to show gratitude by helping others in return. Maybe someone paid for your coffee one day, and you decided to do the same for someone else. Write examples in each ring to honour these moments.

SELF-REFLECTION How many of your good deeds have been inspired by someone else? Do you think you have inspired others to reciprocal kindness? Can gratitude help to build better communities around you?

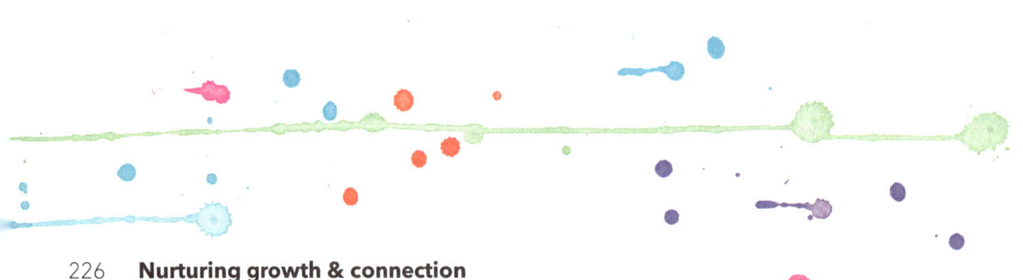

354

The big shift

Try this when
you want to find growth
in struggle

You will need
Paper, watercolours,
paintbrushes, markers

20+ minutes

Think of a challenging situation that you have
overcome, then create a visual representation using
shapes, colours, or forms that show how it felt at the
time. Let this dry, then, using markers, draw a second
layer where you highlight what lessons you learnt
from the experience and how it helped you to grow.

SELF-REFLECTION What are you most thankful for now
that you've overcome the challenge? How does it
feel to sit with discomfort while viewing it through
gratitude? Could you apply this approach to a
current challenge and focus on what it might be
teaching you?

355

Gratitude pause

Try this when
you are faced with a
difficult situation

You will need
Paper, markers, pen, timer

10 minutes

Gratitude doesn't stop difficulties from occurring
in your life, but it helps give you strength to keep
going. When you are faced with a challenging
situation, choose a colour that you feel represents
gratitude and scribble freely on a piece of paper
for 3 minutes. How does gratitude move for you?
Is it slow or fast? Is it circular, linear, or does it have
its own shape? When you've finished, think about
what lessons this challenge might be bringing you.

SELF-REFLECTION Are you someone who quickly
jumps to conclusions? How did it feel to intentionally
pause with gratitude? Did sitting with a positive
emotion shift your perspective on the situation?

356

Gratitude stories

Try this when
you want to explore what
gratitude means to you

You will need
Paper, favourite materials

20+ minutes

Think about stories from your past. What has your family always expressed gratitude for? How have these moments informed your values and way of being? Create an artwork that honours this legacy of appreciation. It might depict a significant life event your family is thankful for, or be an abstract symbol that represents your family's gratitude.

SELF-REFLECTION What has this family legacy taught you about gratitude? Has it helped you grow, or weighed you down? Do your own ideas about gratitude and what you should feel grateful for align with your family's? How do similarities or differences affect your sense of appreciation?

357

Gratitude mask

Try this when
you feel pressured to
be grateful

You will need
Paper plate, markers

20+ minutes

Gratitude can be misused in a society obsessed with relentless positivity. Use a paper plate to create a mask. On the outside of the mask, use symbols to depict the public face of gratitude, showing what false or performative gratitude might look like. You could draw a prison to represent the pressure to be polite or thankful for what you have, which makes you unable to express your needs. On the back of the mask, depict the emotions that gratitude might be covering, such as a sweating face to show guilt, or an angry face for resentment. You can also display any emotions you have suppressed in order to appear grateful.

SELF-REFLECTION Have you ever been pushed to be grateful for something you didn't agree with? Could your gratitude be more connected to external expectations than being personally thankful? How can you stop false gratitude?

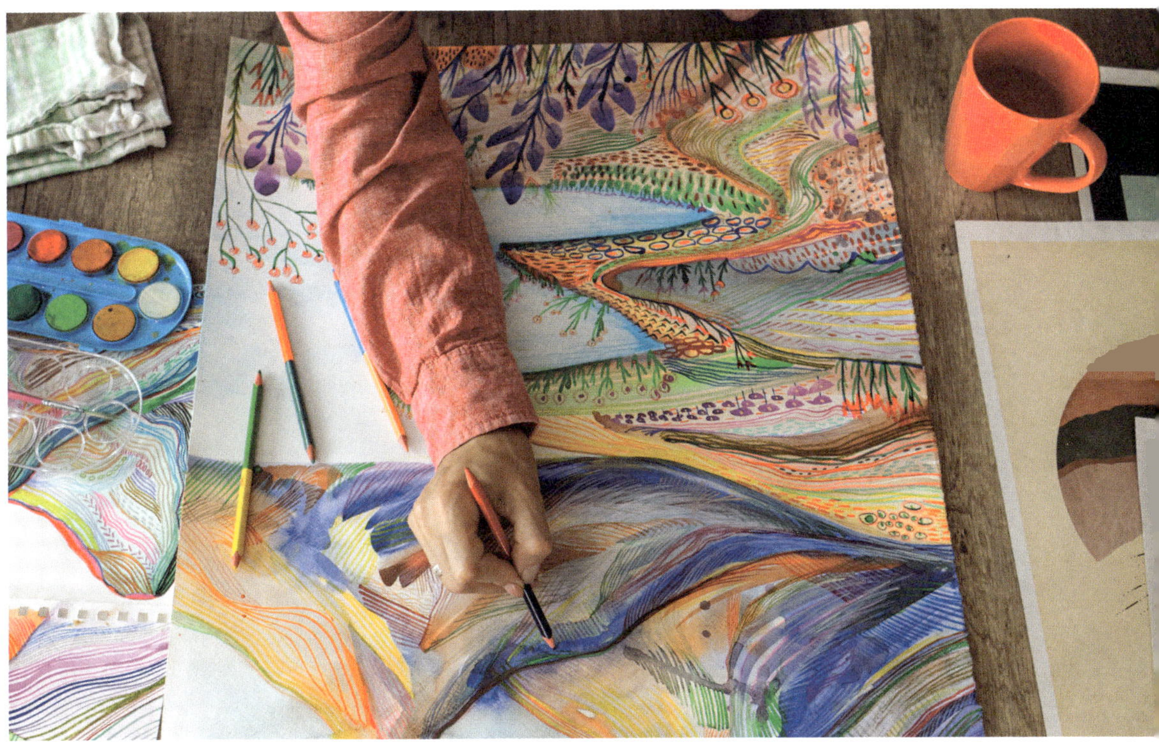

358

Gratitude landscape

Try this when
you want to reflect on
what you value the most

You will need
Paper, favourite materials

20+ minutes

Create a landscape to represent different types of
gratitude. Perhaps include trees that show gratitude
for things you receive, flowers to denote how grateful
you are for what others do for you, and butterflies
or bees to indicate your thanks for the seemingly
effortless magic that happens all around you.

SELF-REFLECTION Does your landscape look realistic
or fake? Are there elements that stand out more than
others? Could this be representing your attitude
towards your own gratitude?

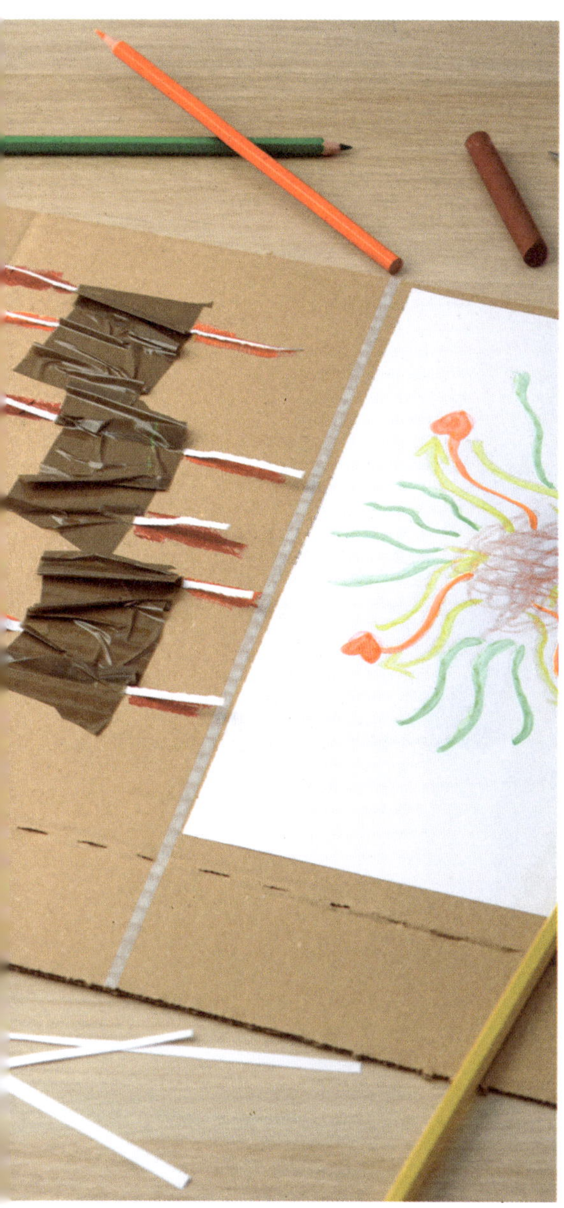

Thanks, but no thanks!

Try this when
you receive unsolicited support

You will need
Cardboard, favourite materials

20+ minutes

Gratitude should stem from within, not be a gesture to please others. There are times when the help we are given might not be what we need in the moment. Divide a piece of cardboard into two. On one side, create an abstract image that represents the good intentions of others and shows your gratitude for them caring. On the other, create an image to express the discomfort of receiving unsolicited help, which perhaps impinges upon your boundaries. You can cut edges or use tape to create rougher textures. When complete, compare both sides and reflect on how they make you feel?

SELF-REFLECTION Will you be able to discern honest gratitude from false in the future? If you have the urge to always be grateful, where does it stem from? Is it useful to be falsely thankful, or do you find it taxing? Sometimes we might need to pretend in order to keep the peace, but don't allow your boundaries to be continually breached.

360

Thank you and...

Try this when
you want to balance
thankfulness with ambition

You will need
Paper, pencil, markers,
coloured pencils

20+ minutes

Draw a circle the size of a grapefruit
in the middle of a piece of paper. Draw
symbols inside it to represent the things
you already have that you are grateful for.
Then draw a circle that surrounds the first
circle, leaving space to add symbols that
represent things that you still wish to
have or accomplish.

SELF-REFLECTION Which circle contains
more symbols? Could there be a way to
balance them out? How did it feel to
integrate satisfaction for what you already
have while also acknowledging that you
still want more?

361

Gratitude circle

Try this when
you want to share your
gratitude with others

You will need
Paper, markers, pen

15+ minutes

Invite one or more close friends or
relatives to start a creative gratitude
journalling practice. Use the exercises in
this chapter as prompts. Gather once a
week or month to share what you are
grateful for. It can be online, in person,
or over a group chat. The objective is to
hold celebration spaces that can bring
peace, connection, and a different
perspective on life.

SELF-REFLECTION Do you enjoy producing
art with others? Could a group like this
help you create a habit of gratitude in
your own life? What difference could you
make in people's lives if you offered this
space for them? Remember, this should
not be a substitute for mental health
services – it should be seen more as a
supportive practice.

Intentional gratitude

If you are struggling to feel grateful, these four exercises might help you to explore and embrace gratitude more fully. This approach can help shift your focus from what's lacking to what supports you.

Try this when
you are ready to embrace gratitude

50 minutes

362 **Just notice**

You will need
Paint, paintbrushes, sponges, cardboard

Start by thinking of something that you are grateful for right now, and choose a colour to represent it. Then, use brushes or sponges to paint the cardboard in this colour, creating a base that you'll use for the other exercises.

363 **Why it matters**

You will need
Coloured paper, scissors, glue, pen

Next, using coloured paper, cut out some geometrical or unstructured shapes. Write about why you chose to be grateful for the thing in the previous exercise on top of them. Paste the cut-outs onto the coloured cardboard base you made.

364 **Underlying feelings**

You will need

Paper, pen, paint, paintbrushes

What feelings are connected to your gratitude? Is it peace, joy, or maybe guilt? Write them all down on a piece of paper and assign a colour to each. Add these colours to the cardboard artwork to represent your emotions, overlapping or highlighting elements in the composition.

365 **Expanding the impact**

You will need

Magazines or image printouts, scissors, glue

Last, using images, illustrate how you can expand this gratitude and share your appreciation with others. Maybe you decide to carry out small acts of kindness or volunteer somewhere? If you aren't sure, allow the images you look through to inspire you.

SELF-REFLECTION Which of the four layers was easier to create? Which was the hardest? Did it help to add meaning and feelings to the gratitude moment? How do you feel about giving back?

Conclusion

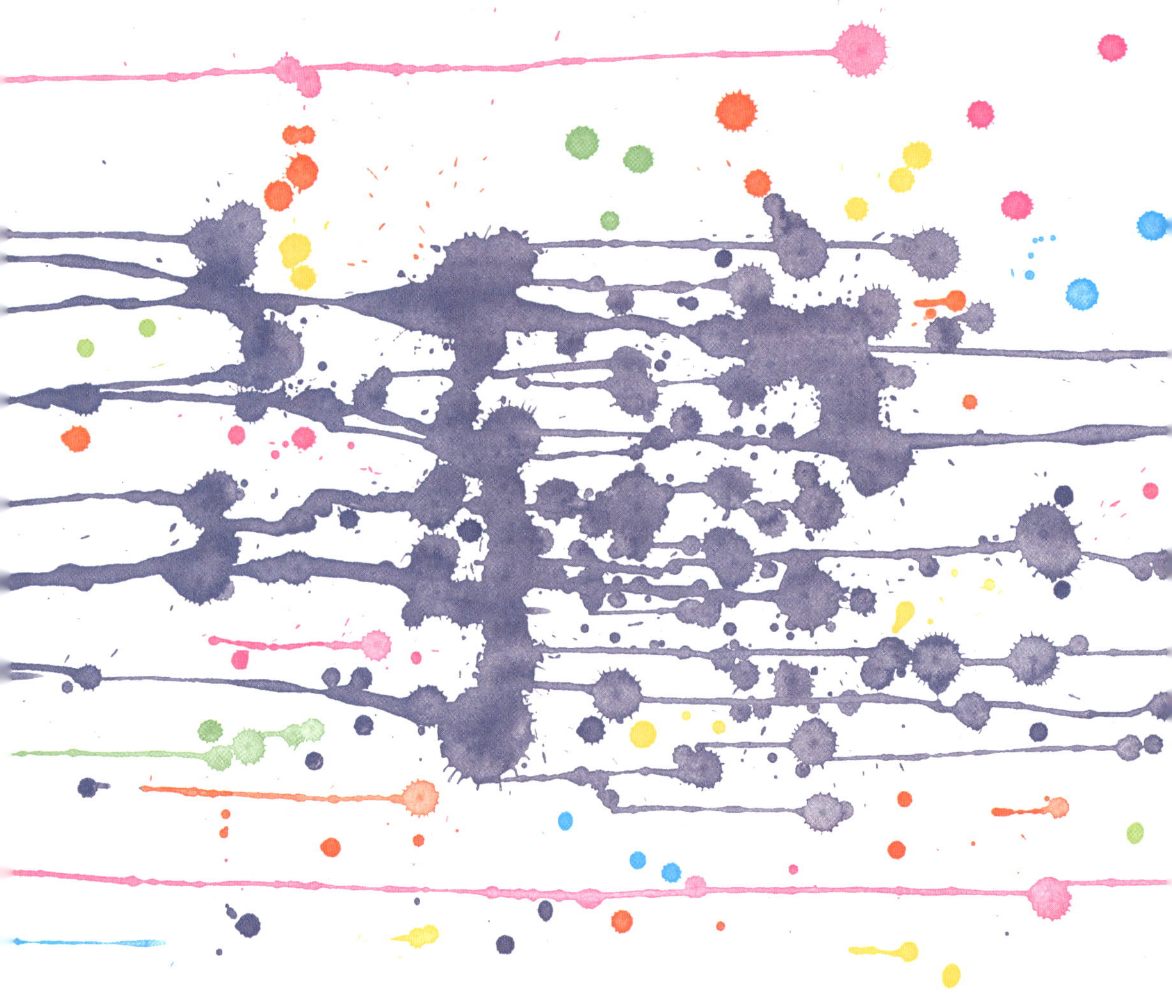

By working through these pages, you will have hopefully reconnected with yourself and begun building a sustainable creative practice that helps you feel better. The ultimate aim of this book is to empower you and your community to care for yourselves with compassion, curiosity, and creativity. Developing these resilience skills allows you to look at yourself and others differently, leading you to a path of self-reflection, growth, and acceptance.

Your life's journey is not about achieving perfection. It is more about being able to manage the tension between perceived failure and personal growth. It's about acknowledging that a never-ending state of happiness isn't realistic, and that negativity will inevitably be a part of your life. You need to reach an equilibrium between the two, and I hope that this book has helped you find a way to sit with both. As you progressed through the different emotional management chapters, you will have learnt that understanding and balancing your feelings – both positive and negative – is crucial, as too much of any emotion can lead to difficulties. The art exercises allow you to connect with your inner wisdom and build trust in your ability to recognize, manage, and express your emotional state. Remember that real growth comes from small daily actions rather than big breakthroughs.

During this journey you might have realized that building gratitude and self-compassion isn't easy. They require patience and courage, but working on them can help you integrate them into your everyday life. You are the writer of your own life story, and you can change the narrative any time you want.

I hope that this book has helped transform your relationship with art, showing that creativity is more than aesthetics – it's a tool for self-reflection, connection, and expression. It also encourages you to nurture yourself and those around you. However, if you have noticed that you are struggling, remember that asking for help or support demonstrates strength and resilience. Reach out to your community, connect with loved ones, or seek the guidance of an art therapist. Healing and living should never be a solo pursuit; it thrives when you feel connected with others.

Index

Acknowledgments

To my family and friends, but especially my husband and son, whose constant love, support, and belief in me have made this book possible. I also want to thank my art therapy and expressive arts therapy colleagues, whose shared vision of preventive and public mental health has helped guide me throughout writing this book in a meaningful and thoughtful way. And lastly, I want to express my deep gratitude to my editors, Jasmin and Kathy, for their insightful feedback, for making me a better writer, and most importantly, for believing in the power of the healing arts and art therapy.

Publisher's Acknowledgments

DK would like to thank Gaynor Sermon for copy-editing, Nigel Wright for photography, Francesco Piscitelli for proofreading, and Ruth Ellis for indexing.

About the author

Nadia Fernanda Paredes Guapo, MA, LMFT 94197, ATR – former President of the American Art Therapy Association (2024–2025) – is a Registered Art Therapist, Licensed Marital and Family Therapist, and Intuition Painting® Facilitator. Nadia helps people connect with their inner creativity and empowers minds and souls through her expressive arts programmes. Her offerings include mindfulness-based programs using embodied arts, art journaling for personal wellness, and international speaking engagements. She hosts a podcast in Spanish called Revolución Creativa, where she shares information about using art as a mental health practice. Nadia is also an art therapy supervisor and adjunct professor at Loyola Marymount University and California Institute of Integral Studies.

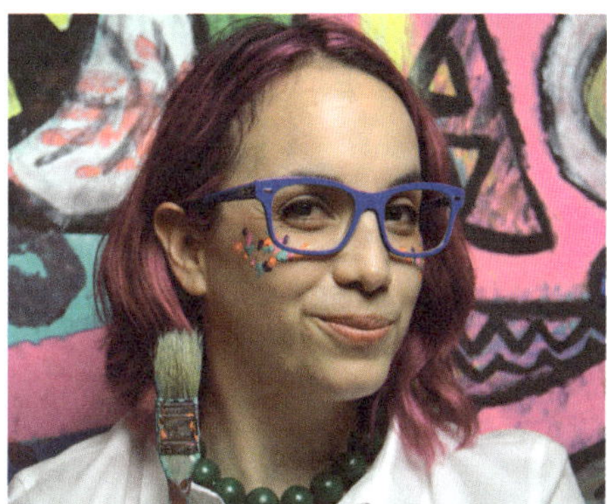

Photography Jesús Vargas Taracena

Picture credits

The publisher would like to thank the following for their kind permission to reproduce their photographs:

(Key: a-above; b-below/bottom; c-centre; f-far; l-left; r-right; t-top)

4 **Getty Images / iStock:** E+ / Frazao Studio Latino (ca). **4-5 Getty Images / iStock:** Netrun78 (c). **6-7 Unsplash:** Dan Cristian Pădure (b). **10-13 Unsplash:** Heather Green (Background). **16 Getty Images / iStock:** E+ / Mixetto (cr); Netrun78 (tr). **19 Getty Images / iStock:** Tomomimo (bl). **20-21 Unsplash:** Heather Green (Background). **23 Unsplash:** Heather Green (Background). **26-27 Unsplash:** Heather Green (Background). **29 Getty Images / iStock:** Happyfoto (b). **34 Unsplash:** Ricardo Viana (tr). **36-37 Unsplash:** Heather Green (Background). **39 Getty Images / iStock:** Fotodaisy (tl). **44 Unsplash:** Heather Green (Background). **50 Getty Images / iStock:** E+ / Supersizer (tr). **55 Unsplash:** Heather Green (Background). **56 Alamy Stock Photo:** Bjarki Reyr (tr). **58-59 Unsplash:** Heather Green (Background). **66 Getty Images / iStock:** E+ / SrdjanPav (tr); Donatas1205 (cr). **68 Unsplash:** Dan Cristian Pădure (t). **73 Nadia Fernanda Paredes Guapo:** (b). **76-77 Unsplash:** Dan Cristian Pădure (t). **78-79 Unsplash:** Heather Green (Background). **83 Unsplash:** Heather Green (Background). **86 Dreamstime.com:** Tuomaslehtinen (tr). **Getty Images / iStock:** Bgwalker (cr). **89 Unsplash:** Dan Cristian Pădure (b). **94-95 Unsplash:** Heather Green (Background). **99 Unsplash:** Heather Green (Background). **103 Dreamstime.com:** Dragonimages (t). **104 Getty Images / iStock:** E+ / Dusan Stankovic (tr). **107 Unsplash:** Heather Green (Background). **108 Getty Images:** Moment / Macbrian Mun (t). **109 Unsplash:** Dan Cristian Pădure (b). **112-113 Getty Images:** Moment / MirageC (t). **114 Unsplash:** Dan Cristian Pădure (t). **117 Getty Images / iStock:** Dusan Stankovic (b). **118-119 Unsplash:** Heather Green (Background). **122 Dreamstime.com:** Trinetuzun (tr). **Getty Images:** Moment / Helder Faria (cr). **124-125 Unsplash:** Heather Green (Background). **127 Unsplash:** Dan Cristian Pădure (t). **128 Getty Images:** Moment / Indie Studios LLC (b). **133 Nadia Fernanda Paredes Guapo:** (tl). **Unsplash:** Dan Cristian Pădure (tr). **137 Unsplash:** Heather Green (Background). **138-139 Getty Images / iStock:** ATHVisions (c). **140 Getty Images:** Moment / Jena Ardell (tr). **Getty Images / iStock:** Vect0r0vich (cr). **142 Unsplash:** Dan Cristian Pădure (t). **146 Getty Images:** Moment / Xiuxia Huang (t). **149 Unsplash:** Dan Cristian Pădure (b). **150 Unsplash:** Heather Green (Background). **153 Getty Images / iStock:** E+ / VeeStudio89 (t). **154-155 Unsplash:** Heather Green (Background). **157 Unsplash:** Dan Cristian Pădure (b). **158 Getty Images:** Moment / Surreal Studios (tr). **161 Getty Images / iStock:** E+ / Miodrag Ignjatovic (b). **162 Getty Images / iStock:** Shisheng Ling (t). **163 Unsplash:** Dan Cristian Pădure (br). **165 Unsplash:** Heather Green (Background). **168 Unsplash:** Dan Cristian Pădure (b). **170-171 Unsplash:** Heather Green (Background). **172 Unsplash:** Dan Cristian Pădure (bl). **173 Dreamstime.com:** Sensay (tr). **176 Getty Images / iStock:** E+ / Edwin Tan (b). **180 Getty Images:** Moment / Nadezda Kozulina (tr). **182 Unsplash:** Dan Cristian Pădure (b). **188 Getty Images / iStock:** Evgenii141 (b). **190-191 Unsplash:** Heather Green (Background). **193 Unsplash:** Dan Cristian Pădure (b). **195 Unsplash:** Heather Green (Background). **197 Shutterstock.com:** Sussi Hj (bl). **198 Getty Images:** Moment / Jane Khomi (tr). **202 Unsplash:** Dan Cristian Pădure (t). **205 Getty Images / iStock:** DigitalVision Vectors / ivetavaicule (b). **206 Unsplash:** Heather Green (Background). **210-211 Unsplash:** Heather Green (Background). **213 Getty Images / iStock:** E+ / Frazao Studio Latino (t). **214 Unsplash:** Dan Cristian Pădure (b). **216 Getty Images / iStock:** DigitalVision Vectors / Pobytov (tr). **218 Unsplash:** Dan Cristian Pădure (bl). **225 Unsplash:** Heather Green (Background). **226 Unsplash:** Dan Cristian Pădure (b). **229 Getty Images:** E+ / Dusan Stankovic (t). **232-233 Unsplash:** Heather Green (Background). **234 Unsplash:** Dan Cristian Pădure. **239 Jesús Vargas Taracena:** (br)

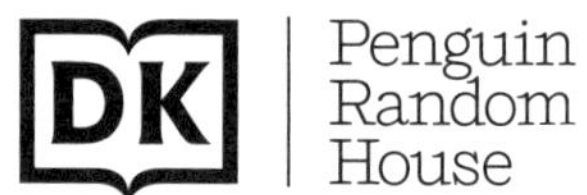

DK LONDON
Editorial Director Zara Anvari
Senior Acquisitions Editor Amy Slack
Editor Jasmin Lennie
Senior Designer Jordan Lambley
Production Editor David Almond
Production Controller Luca Bazzoli
Art Director Maxine Pedliham
Publishing Director Stephanie Jackson

DK DELHI
Picture Research Nishwan Rasool

Design Hello Daly
Editorial Kathy Steer, Gaynor Sermon

First published in Great Britain in 2026 by Dorling Kindersley Limited 20 Vauxhall Bridge Road, London SW1V 2SA

The authorised representative in the EEA is Dorling Kindersley Verlag GmbH. Arnulfstr. 124, 80636 Munich, Germany

Copyright © 2026 Dorling Kindersley Limited
A Penguin Random House Company
10 9 8 7 6 5 4 3 2 1
001–355623–Jan/2026

A CIP catalogue record for this book is available from the British Library.
ISBN: 978-0-2417-8512-6
Printed and bound in China

www.dk.com

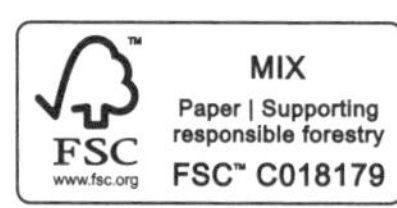